ABORTION:
A WOMAN'S
GUIDE

ABORTION: A WOMAN'S GUIDE

BY

Planned Parenthood of New York City, Inc.

FOREWORD BY

Alan F. Guttmacher, M.D.
President, Planned Parenthood Federation of America, Inc.

Text by Beth Richardson Gutcheon

ABELARD-SCHUMAN, LTD.
New York   London

An Intext Publisher

Library of Congress Cataloging in Publication Data

Gutcheon, Beth Richardson
    Abortion; a woman's guide.

        1. Abortion   2. Conception—Prevention.
I. Planned Parenthood of New York City.   II. Title.
[DNLM: 1. Abortion, Induced—Popular works. WQ225 G983a 1973]
RG734.G87 1973   613.9'43   72-9549
ISBN 0-200-04003-0
ISBN 0-200-04008-1 (pbk.)

Illustrations by Judy A. Skorpil

Photographs by Camera Arts

Abelard-Schuman Limited, 257 Park Avenue South, New York N.Y. 10010

Published on the same day in Canada by Longman Canada Limited.

Library of Congress Catalogue Card Number:72-9549
Printed in the United States of America

Typography by S. S. Drate

Acknowledgments

I am indebted to various staff members of Planned Parenthood of New York City for the help and cooperation they gave in the preparation of this book.

The suggestions, factual information and critical comments of Alfred F. Moran, Mrs. Jane Johnson, Mrs. Elizabeth Roman, Mrs. Merna Friedman, Miss Corinne Schreider, and Dr. Sherwin Kaufman were invaluable.

I wish to thank also the staff at Planned Parenthood of New York City's 22nd Street Center, upon whose work so much of this book is based.

Finally, I should like to express my gratitude for the continuing editorial and substantive help of Mrs. Marcia Lawrence and Ira L. Neiger, co-directors of PPNYC's Public Information and Education Department.

B.R.G.

Contents

This book is dedicated to Jane Roe,
Mary Doe, and to all the others, both
women and men, who helped make
abortion legal and safe in the United
States.

Foreword

Four hundred years ago, François Mauriceau, the most eminent obstetrician of the Early Renaissance, likened maternity to a great uncharted sea full of dangerous shoals upon which the ship of pregnancy frequently foundered. In the intervening years, medical map makers have well charted that sea so that few shoals threaten. This *Woman's Guide* succeeds in doing the same for abortion.

The *Guide* speaks to the individual patient like a concerned, empathetic, knowledgeable friend. It begins by discussing her psychological and physical reactions to the suspicion of pregnancy. It then guides her through its diagnosis and supports her through in-depth counseling during the difficult decision-making period by clearly spelling out the multiple options open to her. It also catalogues for her the many conscious and sub-conscious factors that lead to unplanned pregnancy in this contraceptive age, with the hope that by under-standing the genesis of her own behavior she might prevent the repetition of unplanned pregnancy. The fac-tual step-by-step account of what is involved in the induction of early and late abortion should be of great importance to anyone undergoing such an operation. Since one of the most important antidotes to fear is knowledge, the *Guide* is a valuable antidote. Inclusion of an extensive discussion of contraception is well merited.

It is heartening to realize that now, after January, 1973, more than half of the 3.8 billion people of the world reside in political jurisdictions where abortion is permitted not only for medical but for sociological rea-sons as well. Liberalization of abortion is a rapidly pro-gressing socio-legal phenomenon; it can not and will not be stopped until it is global in application.

Abortion: A Woman's Guide should be of tremendous value to individuals in need of knowledge and advice. Its simple and humane approach to the problem of abortion cannot help but put the procedure in proper perspective for the general public.

Alan F. Guttmacher, M.D.

1

Facing It

Your period is late.

Well, there is nothing unusual in that, you tell yourself. You just need a good night's sleep, or maybe you're catching a cold.

After a few days, you say, "It's late because I'm anxious." You try to think about something else. You try so hard you can hardly bring yourself to wake up in the morning; as long as you stay asleep you don't have to think about anything at all. "I'm exhausted," you say. "That's why it's late."

After a week has gone by, it begins to look as if your period is not just late, it is altogether absent.

Even that is not *so* unusual. You have heard of many women who have skipped periods completely during times of stress or illness. Maybe you begin to search your memory for other things you have heard—about hot baths that bring on delayed menstruation, about running up five flights of stairs, jumping off porches, taking laxatives. But mixed in with the hearsay and old wives' tales, you cannot quite force out of your mind one hard fact.

If you had intercourse last month, the odds are more than even that you are pregnant.

This is somehow unthinkable if you have not planned to be pregnant, and especially if you have never been pregnant before. It is *your* body, known, familiar; you realize in an abstract way that it is equipped for pregnancy, but the idea that it should suddenly begin to function in this strange and unfamiliar way without your willing or intending it seems utterly unreasonable. How can it happen to you?

Hoping to discover signs that it has not happened—perhaps a twinge of pre-menstrual cramps—you may instead start to notice nausea or a slight swelling or tenderness in your breasts. You may observe that you are reacting in an unaccustomed way to certain foods —suddenly onions give you heartburn. Or you may have a middle-of-the-night yearning for tomato juice or Chinese food—even for something you usually hate. Odd cravings are unusual so soon; but as if to add insult to injury, an unplanned pregnancy often has the most intense early symptoms, because of the woman's emotional tension. On the other hand, symptoms may not be present at all. Certainly presence or absence proves nothing; you might be sick as a dog from no other cause than your worry.

These days can be some of the rockiest of a woman's life. They always have been. Over the centuries, women faced with unwanted pregnancies have been known to maim and even kill themselves in attempts to put their lives back to what they were before that first missed period. They have swallowed powerful medicines or actual poisons; they have hoped that by douching with caustic solutions or sticking foreign objects into the uterus they could physically force their organs to do what they desperately wanted them to do. But these measures *never* help—and they frequently result in serious injury, sterility, or death.

At this point, there is only one thing that *can* help. To relieve your tension and put you back in control of your life, you need to find out for sure if you really are pregnant or not.

And the only way to do that is to wait two weeks from the day your period was due—because it takes that long for pregnancy to be physically detectable—and then get a medical pregnancy diagnosis: not just a test done on your urine, but an internal examination of your uterus, via the vagina, performed by a doctor.

Getting Pregnancy Diagnosed

This is a very difficult step for a good many women. It means sharing your problem with someone else, which is painful enough; and sharing it with a doctor, who is the last person some women feel like turning to. There are also women who feel that knowing they are pregnant won't do them any good—that all their alternatives are equally humiliating and terrifying. Other women are boggled simply because they have no idea whom to call or where to go. Some unmarried women put off going for a test because they feel defensive or

guilty about the sexual activity that caused their pregnancy. Some who are very young are afraid that anyone
they ask for help will report it to their parents or schools
or employers.

But hard as it may seem to let an outsider know you
could be pregnant, it's a lot worse not to know yourself.

And though an unwanted pregnancy is clearly a crisis
in any woman's life, no matter who she is, things are not
nearly as bad as they were two years ago, or ten; and
with the U.S. Supreme Court's ruling in January, 1973,
they have come a long, long way indeed from what your
grandmother faced.

First, there are alternatives available to you, of which
legal abortion is now firmly one, wherever you live in
the United States.

Second, wherever you live, you can get help in coping
with the alternatives. A telephone call, local or long
distance, will put you in touch with either of two nonprofit organizations with nationwide networks of services. They are not peddling any private line of hooey;
they don't want to judge you or pressure you; they don't
want to talk you into anything or out of anything. What
they *will* do is explain to you exactly what your options
are and give you whatever facts you need to make your
decision.

The *Clergy Consultation Service on Abortion* has
offices in 34 states and individual clergymen and clergy-
women (plus non-clergy associates) in all other states.
Clergy services do not include pregnancy testing or
referrals for it. But once you know for sure that you are
pregnant, you can call them for professional help in
sorting out your feelings, so that you can decide what
to do about your pregnancy; and if your decision is

abortion, they will refer you to a doctor, clinic, or hospital that will serve you.

The other agency is *Planned Parenthood*, which deals with the whole range of family planning services—contraception, pregnancy detection, abortion, voluntary sterilization, infertility treatment, and prenatal care. There are 188 Planned Parenthood affiliates in 43 states and the District of Columbia, and they operate some 700 medical clinics. Besides contraception, which all of them provide, many of the clinics do pregnancy testing and some have even more comprehensive services, including abortion. But any Planned Parenthood affiliate, whether it actually provides a particular service or not, will tell you where and how you can get it, and will answer medical or legal questions if you have them. If you are a minor, or if you are worried about your ability to pay, they will advise you how to proceed. If you feel you need a professional counselor, they will either have one on staff or refer you to one.

Information and referral are free from both Planned Parenthood and the Clergy Consultation Service, and there is a listing of their local offices and phone numbers at the end of this book.

Maybe you already have a doctor you know and like and feel you can discuss a possible pregnancy with. Going to a private doctor for a pregnancy test is the most expensive way of getting one, but if the money won't be an extra source of anxiety, you might be most comfortable in private, familiar surroundings. But if you feel uneasy about calling the doctor—if you are afraid he will tell your family, or hassle you about your sex life, or try to influence your decision about the pregnancy—for heaven's sake, don't go to him just because you always have before. Ethically, it's none of his business what you decide; nor is it his business to tell anyone else. On the other hand, if you are a minor and/or married, he may be skittish about treating you without the consent or, at any rate, knowledge of a parent, guardian, or husband. There may be a local law regulating this or he thinks there is, or it is the standard practice locally, or maybe it is just his own policy. If you aren't sure of the laws in your area or the attitude of your doctor, consider calling Planned Parenthood if only to be referred to a doctor you *can* be sure of.

If money is a problem or if you just don't want to go to a private doctor, many hospitals have free or low-cost family planning clinics where you can arrange for a pregnancy test. To find out about them, call the main number of a hospital near you and ask to speak to the nurse in charge of the family planning clinic. You will need to ask her when and where the clinic meets, whether you need to "pre-register," how much it will cost, what area the clinic serves (sometimes you have to live in a certain neighborhood to be eligible), and if anyone's consent besides your own is required to get treatment. It is also a good idea to ask whether the hospital gives tests for venereal disease, and if so how they notify you of the results.

Another possibility is to call the Health Department, which is listed in the phone book, and tell them you want a pregnancy test. They will either be able to provide one themselves or refer you to a hospital that will do it on their behalf. This will probably be free, but ask about cost anyway, and about consents and the VD test.

Up until December, 1972, it was also possible to drop into the corner drug store and pick up something advertised as a handy do-it-yourself pregnancy testing kit. At that point, however, the Federal Food and Drug Administration ordered the recall of the Ova II kits on the grounds that they were "inaccurate, unreliable and prone to give false results"; thus it is fairly unlikely that you are going to run across this particular home chemistry set now.

Then again, you may. Or other manufacturers may decide to put other urine-testing products on the market, since they know as well as anybody else that, of course, you would rather be able to learn if you are pregnant or not without letting anyone know; and that for a few women, getting to a doctor may be a real logistical problem. Maybe such kits will be improved, made easier to use and more accurate than those now banned. But even if they were to match the reliability of a professional laboratory test, you are still going to have to see a doctor—because any urine test provides only half the information needed to be sure that a pregnancy exists or that it doesn't.

How Pregnancy Is Detected

After conception has occurred, a woman's body begins to produce a special hormone called chorionic gonadotropin; and normally, by the time a missed period is ten days to two weeks overdue, enough of the hormone has accumulated in her system to show up in her urine. Occasionally, though, the accumulation process requires more time, and there are conditions that can cause the hormone to be present when a pregnancy is not.

On the other hand, if a woman really is pregnant, some other changes in her body should also have begun to take place by now. The vaginal tissues will have turned slightly bluish in color; the uterus will have become a little larger and more cushiony to the doctor's touch when he examines you internally. So if the condition of the uterus and vagina is compatible with the test results, and with what you have told the doctor about the date of the last normal menstrual period you actually had, then he can make a definite diagnosis.

If you have not been keeping careful track of your periods, you may not be sure of the exact date the last one started, but it is important, particularly if you are thinking about an abortion. Look back, maybe there is some event you can tie it to. Perhaps you remember wanting to do something special that cramps interfered with, or you were dressing in a rush—to get to class or work or to take the baby for a checkup—just as you discovered you had spotted your last clean pair of drawers. Anyway, however you work it out, do it as closely as you can before you go for your medical examination.

When you call the doctor, hospital, or clinic to make your appointment for the examination, you will be given instructions about the urine sample. You may be asked to bring with you a container of "first urine"— more highly concentrated chemically, because it is produced the first thing in the morning before you have eaten or drunk anything—or you may simply be asked to give a sample when you arrive for the examination. Some doctors will ask you to drop a sample off at the laboratory a few days before your appointment.

For the internal examination, you will be asked to take off your clothes and drape a sheet or a paper gown around yourself. Then, in the doctor's examining room, you will lie on your back on a high couch-table with your hips at the end of the table and your feet up, resting on metal supports called stirrups, so that your knees are bent.

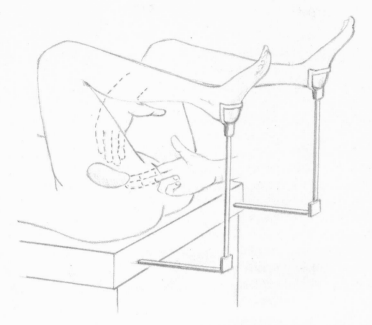

In a pelvic examination, the doctor inserts two fingers of his
gloved hand, lubricated with a jelly, into the vagina and places
his other hand on the lower abdomen.

First, the doctor will want to see your vagina and
your cervix—the neck of the uterus. To accomplish this,
he will insert a metal instrument called a speculum into
the vagina, to spread and hold its walls apart. Since the
speculum is usually cold, this is not the world's most
delightful experience, but it is not painful. Just relax
your muscles, and the speculum will go in as easily as
a tampon.

The doctor will probably then do a Pap test. This has
nothing to do with diagnosing pregnancy; it is a procedure for detecting cancer of the cervix. But every
woman is well advised to have it done at least once every

year, and most doctors do it routinely whenever they are in the cervical neighborhood. It involves taking a smear of mucus from the cervix by touching it lightly with a little cotton swab on a stick, like a long Q-Tip, and transferring the smear to a glass slide for processing. All this takes about a minute, after which the speculum is removed.

Next, the doctor determines the size and feel of the uterus with a bimanual examination. He inserts two fingers of one hand into the vagina so that he can touch the cervix, he places his other hand on the abdomen, and he feels the shape and size of the uterus between the fingers of the two hands. Again, this is not precisely comfortable, but the internal hand is gloved and well lubricated, and there is certainly no pain.

If the urine test is negative and other evidence inconclusive at this point, the doctor may suggest that you wait a week, then come back and go through the whole process all over again if you still haven't menstruated. Or he may offer you a dose of progesterone—pills or an injection. Progesterone makes some people feel pretty horrible, but if you are indeed not pregnant, it will bring on your period. If it does not, at least your uncertainty will be over; its failure is a virtually sure sign of pregnancy.

No such delay may be necessary, though. All the evidence may immediately indicate pregnancy, and the doctor will tell you so. He will also tell you how many weeks along you are, which may be more than you thought. He will start counting, not from the date of conception, presumed or even known, but from the start of your last menstrual period—because this is the very last day on which it can be said for sure that you were nonpregnant. So if you normally menstruate at fairly regular 28-day intervals and were two weeks overdue at the time of your examination, according to this formula you are six weeks pregnant.

Now That You Know

Once the pregnancy has been officially confirmed, you are bound to experience some mixed feelings, to put it mildly. Some of the tug-of-war comes from all the conflicting taboos and totems about what you ought to feel: you *ought* to be thrilled, you *ought* to be grateful, you *ought* to be ashamed, you *ought* to be punished. But it also comes from what you really *do* feel, and one of the miracles of pregnancy is that it is possible to respond to it quite genuinely with total ambivalence. You can be glad about it and want it ended at the same time with equal intensity. You may feel angry, frightened, outraged; yet somewhere in your heart of hearts you may also feel a little flicker of pride, even relief. Your body has fulfilled an important function, whether you like it or not, and however much you may not want to be pregnant at this moment in your life, it is good to know that you can be—that everything works, already or still.

But you may now be discovering that you are a little muddled about *how* everything works. Even if you have been pregnant before and especially if you have not, there are apt to be gaps in your knowledge; and it is not necessarily any comfort to realize that almost every other adult's information is equally shaky.

If you would like to fill in some of the gaps, that is what the next few pages are for. If you already know as much about conception as you care to learn, feel free to skip.

How Conception Occurs

One thing everybody is pretty clear on is that conception is the result of sexual intercourse, when an egg in a woman's body is joined by a sperm from a man's body.

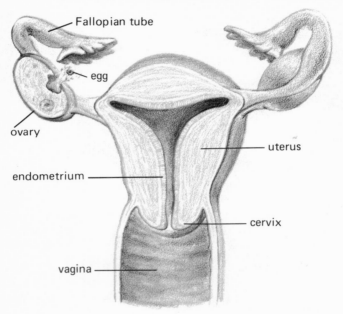

Female reproductive organs.

When a woman is born she has in her body all the eggs, or ova, her body will release throughout her lifetime. They repose in an immature state in the ovaries, which are small organs lying outside the uterus, adjacent to the Fallopian tubes. These two tubes extend like fat, pink morning glories from the uterus to the ovaries, and once a month one or the other acts as a conduit to pass a single egg from an ovary to the uterus.

The uterus is a small hollow organ like an upside-

down pear, about three or four inches long in a nonpregnant woman. If an egg is fertilized, the uterus becomes
its environment; it is where the fertilized egg develops
into an embryo and then a fetus, and where the fetus
remains until gestation is completed, unless the pregnancy is terminated. At the bottom of the uterus is the
cervix, or neck, which contains a small opening.

The cervix protrudes slightly into the vagina, the
corridor connecting your internal reproductive organs
with the outside world. Relaxed, the walls of the vagina
touch, but the space between is capable of great expan-
sion—to accommodate the penis during intercourse and
the baby passing from the uterus during birth. Outside
the vagina are the external genitals, or vulva.

When a girl reaches puberty—usually somewhere between her twelfth and fifteenth birthdays—her reproductive organs are physically mature. They then begin
a cycle of activity that will continue, month after
month, for thirty or thirty-five years, except during
pregnancy.

The cycle starts when a certain hormone produced in
the pituitary gland (located at the base of the brain) sets
a chain of events in motion in the ovaries. First, several
follicles in the ovaries, each containing an egg, begin to
grow larger while the others remain dormant. As they
grow, the follicles release another hormone, estrogen.
This causes the lining of the uterus to thicken so that
if an egg should be fertilized it will find a soft, nourish-
ing surface in which to implant itself.

The follicles grow for about seven days, at which
point one begins to outstrip the rest. It continues to
swell and develop, while the others slowly regress to
their former state. (Occasionally, more than one egg
will develop and be released and fertilized, causing

twins. Such twins have different genes and are not identical; identical twins occur when a single egg divides in
two after fertilization.)

The largest follicle goes on growing for another couple of days or so. Then, about the fourteenth day of the
cycle, the follicle ruptures and releases the egg. This is
called ovulation.

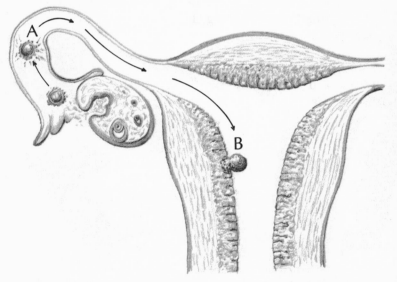

Passage of an egg (shown greatly enlarged) from the Fallopian
tube into the uterus. At point A, egg is fertilized by sperm. At
point B, it attaches itself to the wall of the uterus.

At once, the egg is drawn into a Fallopian tube, down
which it will travel to the uterus; and if fertilization is
going to occur it will happen here—in the tube—within
twenty-four to thirty-six hours after ovulation. Beyond
that time, the egg is no longer fresh, and fertilization is
virtually impossible.

If it has not occurred, there is no more need for a

thickened uterine lining, so the hormone level drops. This sends a message back to the pituitary gland to start the next cycle, which begins with menstrual bleeding to wash away the unused lining and the unfertilized egg. At the same time, new follicles begin to grow.

Confusingly, although fertilization can only take place during one twenty-four- to thirty-six-hour period in each menstrual cycle, this does not mean that *intercourse* must occur during these hours for pregnancy to result.

When a man ejaculates during intercourse, he releases into the vagina a milky fluid called semen, containing hundreds of millions of sperm which can live in the woman's body for at least two or three days. They travel very rapidly through the cervix, through the uterus and into the Fallopian tubes, where they may be present when the egg is released even though intercourse took place days before. Similarly, even if intercourse occurs as much as a day after ovulation, the sperm travel so swiftly that conception can still occur.

Even so, that does seem to leave twenty-four days out of a typical twenty-eight-day cycle when you are "safe" —when sperm and egg cannot possibly get together. Unfortunately, not every cycle is a nice predictable twenty-eight days with ovulation firmly in the middle. Ovulation is triggered by a hormonal buildup in your system that may be unusually quick one month or unusually slow the next, so the best that can be said is only that there are certain days—such as during menstruation—when you are least likely to get pregnant; you are never really "safe." Conception *can* occur on any day of the month, even during your period, for an egg *can* be released at any time.

Maybe you have heard that douching immediately

after intercourse washes away sperm before they can enter the uterus. Not so; sperm move too fast for any douche, no matter what you use.

Nor does it make any difference what position you use for lovemaking. If the penis enters the vagina, pregnancy is possible. Even if a man withdraws his penis before ejaculation, some semen may be released into the vagina or just outside it, and sperm may still find their way into the tubes—because sperm travel by themselves, they don't have to be jet-propelled.

Home-made condoms like Baggies or Saran Wrap, covering the penis during intercourse, will be no more reliable. They are not nearly strong enough and cannot possibly cover completely enough to capture *all* the sperm released; and if even a few drops are spilled during ejaculation or when the penis is withdrawn, that's plenty.

You may also have heard that you cannot conceive as long as you are breast-feeding, and up to a point, it is true. Breast-feeding a baby does provide the mother with some natural protection against pregnancy. But it is only for a short period, perhaps up to six weeks. It does *not* protect her for the duration of the baby's nursing, as many a woman has learned the hard way.

What Happens Now?

If you have become pregnant as a result of trusting any of these non-methods of birth control, you certainly don't lack for company.

On the other hand, it may be that you already understood quite well how conception occurs, and that you were faithfully using one of the most reliable methods of contraception. If so, you probably feel especially angry and let down at this point, and no one could blame you. It's bad enough to be caught when you're taking chances, but to be caught when you're being as careful as you can be is one of life's really bitter experiences. And yet, as you know, there are no guarantees—unless you avoid intercourse altogether, there are still no *totally* sure methods of avoiding pregnancy. At this point in medical history, every act of lovemaking involves some risk of conception to a woman in her fertile years, if only a fraction of a percent.

Anyway, whatever you did or didn't do before, your immediate concern has to be what you can do now; and few women faced with an unwanted pregnancy find it simple or easy to know what they want to do. However sure you are that you want an abortion, there are going to be moments when you will doubt and cross-examine yourself, just as there are going to be moments of anguish and resentment if you decide to complete the pregnancy.

Decision-making is a whole complicated subject that needs and will get a chapter to itself. Where you get a pregnancy test probably doesn't matter much as long as you get one; but how you make your decision, and how wisely, will have repercussions for the rest of your life. If you are lucky, you will have a husband, friend, or family to stand by you. But you may not; and even if you do you may find that you need more specific information or more professional support than they can give. At this critical moment in your life, it will be especially important for you to remember there are agencies to turn to that believe you have the ability and the right to decide what to do, and that your freedom to exercise choice about your future is precious.

2

Decision-Making

A woman who is unexpectedly pregnant has three alternatives open to her. She can have the baby and keep it. She can have the baby and surrender it—temporarily, to foster care, pending a change in circumstances; or permanently, to adoption. Or she can have an abortion.

Probably these three possibilities have swum in and out of your head from the moment you first missed your period. You confront them head-on on the day you learn for sure that you are pregnant. You must make a decision quickly, and you must make it under enormous pressure. To do this, you need practical information and you need to understand and trust yourself.

Getting a legal abortion is a relatively new option for

most women in the United States, so the chances are that you have less information about this alternative than about the others. Some women may be unaware that it is an option for them at all. But it has been specifically defined as your right by the United States Supreme Court, and the decision to have an abortion or not have it is up to you. State laws still differ, but there has been enough change in enough states for a legal abortion to be within the reach of almost any woman, rich or poor, if it is her choice. If it is not yet available locally, you may have to travel—to a nearby state or even to one that is not so near. Nevertheless, the option is there.

If you are going to consider it, one of the first things you may want to know is what it involves physically.

Embryo at sixth week of pregnancy. This is its actual size.

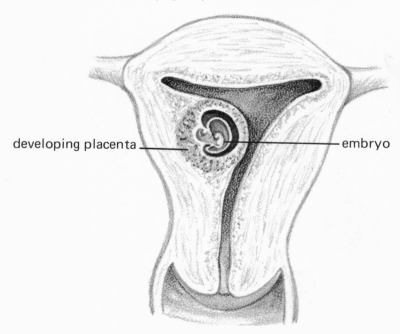

developing placenta   embryo

The Medical Facts

After an egg is fertilized, it continues to drift down the Fallopian tube; and by about the twentieth day of the cycle, it implants itself in the wall of the uterus. It has been there for about a week by the time you start looking for your period, and by the time another two weeks have gone by, its presence is medically detectable. At this point, the sixth week of pregnancy, the embryo is a tiny bump about half an inch long on the inner wall of the uterus.

Embryo at tenth week of pregnancy. This is its actual size.

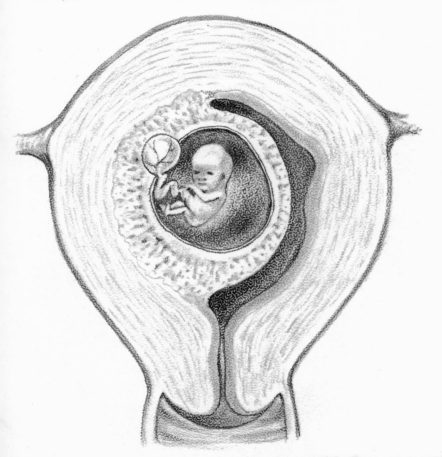

Between the sixth week and the tenth, the embryo grows about an inch. It is connected to the uterine wall and is surrounded by a bag filled with fluid. The bag is made of thin tissue called amniotic membranes, and the liquid, which acts as a cushion for the embryo, is called amniotic fluid. All around the outside of the amniotic sac, placenta is developing. This is a mass of tissue which provides nourishment to the embryo. At ten weeks the entire bulk of material—embryo, amniotic fluid, and placenta—is about the size of a plum.

Up to the twelfth week, this material can be mechanically removed by one of two simple procedures. The traditional one is called Dilation and Curettage—for short, D & C. The opening in the cervix is gradually *dilated*—stretched—until it is wide enough to accept a *curette,* a rod-shaped instrument with a sort of sharp-edged spoon on the end. The doctor inserts the curette into the uterus and gently scrapes the walls clean.

The second method, which is the one more commonly used now, is called suction, vacuum aspiration, or vacuum curettage. The cervix is dilated, and a slender hollow tube is inserted into the uterus. The tube is connected to a small vacuum pump, and low suction empties the uterus. This is generally followed by a final cleanup with a small curette.

Both the D & C and suction procedures take less than ten minutes and can be performed under a local anesthetic—you don't have to be put to sleep.

Between the tenth and the fourteenth weeks of the pregnancy, the embryo doubles in size. The amount of fluid in the amniotic sac increases, and the placenta grows larger as the flow of blood to it increases. This causes the walls of the uterus to stretch and become quite soft and thin, so that after the twelfth week insertion of a curette or suction tube is risky. By the fourteenth week, the embryo has become a fetus and is too large to be removed from the uterus by D & C or suction without great pain to the patient and possible damage to the uterus.

If the circumstances warrant, a few places will sometimes do a D & C or suction procedure between the twelfth and fourteenth weeks of pregnancy; but between the fourteenth and sixteenth weeks, there is no medically accepted method of performing an abortion. This two-to-four-week period is called the interim period. If you have reached it at the time you decide to seek an abortion, you will probably be advised to wait until you reach the sixteenth week, when it is possible to do a saline abortion.

A saline abortion, often called "salting out," is performed in a hospital, usually between the sixteenth and twentieth weeks of pregnancy. With a long hypodermic needle inserted into the uterus through the abdomen, a doctor removes some of the fluid from the amniotic sac and replaces it with a solution of salt and water. Some time later (the waiting period lasts from five hours to two days) the uterus begins to contract, as in labor. Contractions continue until the uterus pushes out the fetal and placental material.

This procedure should not be performed before the sixteenth week, because before that time the amniotic sac may not be large enough for the doctor to locate it easily with the needle. The saline method carries about seven times more risk of complications than early abortion and is unquestionably more expensive. But if it is necessary to do an abortion after the twelfth week of pregnancy, salting out is the safest method available and is the way about 95 percent of all late abortions are done.

Complicated though all this may seem, the medical

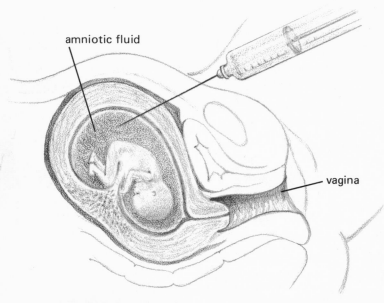

amniotic fluid

vagina

A saline abortion. A needle is inserted through the abdominal wall, and some of the amniotic fluid will be removed and replaced with a saline solution.

aspects of abortion are relatively easy to grasp and consider, compared to the emotional questions that go with them. To a certain extent you may fear the physical pain involved or you may worry about the small but undeniable risks involved in submitting to this or any surgical procedure. But these factors are not really likely to be what bothers you most—continuing a pregnancy involves actually greater medical risk than an abortion, and childbirth is certain to involve some degree of physical pain.

For most women, the real problem is more likely to

be that even though they really did not want to have a baby, they *did* want to become pregnant. Or they wanted the experience of giving birth without wanting or being able to keep and raise a child. Or even if they wholeheartedly wanted and tried to prevent conception, now that it has taken place, they feel a sense of responsibility or protectiveness toward the pregnancy as much as they feel the imperative need to terminate it.

The Emotional Pulls

Many medical and social workers in the field of family planning have come to feel that there is almost no such thing as a totally unwanted pregnancy. No matter what we feel about our sexual activity, no matter how we respond to the notion of having a child, something in us as women—in our minds, our hearts, our glands, our wombs—seems to welcome the fact of being pregnant. As a result, no matter how firmly a woman feels that abortion is the best choice for her, she almost surely will also feel some resistance to the idea, consciously or unconsciously. And if she is not aware that this ambivalence is totally natural, she can let it build in her until she feels she is being torn apart.

She may feel intensely, for the sake of her whole future and the future of everybody she loves most—of children she already has or children she might have in the future—that she does not want to continue her pregnancy.

Yet she may feel just as strongly that she does want to continue it, or that she ought to want to; and feeling so, she wonders if abortion is indeed the right thing, or

even if there is something selfish or unnatural or unwomanly in seeking an abortion. Being pregnant makes
her feel like a woman. What does wanting to terminate
the pregnancy make her?

There are lots of answers to that question. It can be
said that continuing a pregnancy can be as selfish an act
as ending it. It can be said that ending a pregnancy that
threatens everything that makes a woman's life worth
living is no more unnatural than treating an illness that
can cripple her. It can also be said that when a woman
makes informed and intelligent decisions concerning
her own fertility, she is performing the most womanly
function of all.

But ultimately the only person who can really answer
these questions—the only person who has the right to
—is the woman involved, for herself. Other people can
provide information and advice, but the most important
factors in your decision are within you. They have to do
with who you are, your expectations of yourself and
your future, your religious and ethical beliefs, your feelings about abortion, your financial situation and family
setup, and the individual set of circumstances and moti-
vations that resulted in your pregnancy. Having examined these factors, you can then make what you feel will
be the most positive and responsible choice for *you*.

This is not to say that reaching a decision will au-
tomatically cause all doubts and confusion to melt
away. But truly and honestly confronting yourself, sorting through the motives and emotions that cause you
confusion, and understanding why you became pregnant—this can help you be sure your decision is right.
And that conviction is important, not only because you
will have to live with your decision, whatever it is, for
the rest of your life; but also because it will help you to

trust yourself and your strength and ability to make decisions for yourself in the future.

Why Women Become Pregnant

A good case can be made that it is not really lack of information about contraception that makes for unplanned pregnancies as much as it is a lack of information about our own motives. There are very few women who are honestly unaware that pregnancy results from intercourse. And most women are aware, at least to some degree, that there are methods and devices that help to prevent conception.

Why, then, do so many women find themselves pregnant without deliberately, consciously choosing to be?

Some women certainly would like to have contraceptive information or devices, but they don't know where to get them or they're afraid to ask for them. Perhaps they are afraid that because of age or marital status they will encounter unpleasantness if they try to get contraceptive help in their own communities; maybe they know very well they will be hassled. Anyway, they choose to take a chance.

Some women may be using contraception, but the method fails. Not every woman finds it possible to use the most effective methods. Maybe the Pill causes a woman unpleasant side effects, or the idea of putting a diaphragm inside herself disturbs her, or she doesn't think full-time protection like the Pill or the IUD is necessary for the tempo of her sexual activity. She may feel she has to rule out all prescription methods because they require going to a doctor. Or she prefers to leave contraception to the man, who promises to withdraw in time but fails, or who holds off putting on a condom till too late. Maybe he tells her he was sterilized, but he wasn't; that happens, too. Anyway, again, you might say she has chosen to take a chance—or that she was forced to.

If you are in either of these groups, you may find in examining your feelings that one of them is anger against the circumstances that prevented you from protecting yourself better. You may also have other conflicting emotions about your pregnancy now that it is a fact. But if you feel you sincerely did not want to become pregnant, then you should trust that conviction. The point of examining your motives is not to see if your pregnancy is somehow your fault, something to blame yourself for, but to discover if there is something in yourself that really wanted and needed to become pregnant; and if so, if that same drive has anything to do with a real desire or need to have a baby, for there are many situations in which the two can be clearly separated.

Often a woman knows about effective At-the-Time contraception and uses it regularly, yet chooses not to use it on a particular occasion. Maybe a sexual situation that was just too good to miss came up at a time when no contraceptive was handy; maybe she deliberately decided that to stop in the middle of making love would ruin the moment. That's a clear choice, and often your sexual desires can override your feelings about getting pregnant.

On the other hand, if a woman repeatedly chooses not to use contraception when she just as easily, or almost as easily, could use it, there may be other factors at work. For one thing, sex is rarely so consistently ecstatic that you cannot possibly tear yourself away for thirty seconds, considering what's at stake. But to think in quite such a logical way about taking precautions, you must have a fairly logical, straightforward attitude towards sex to begin with, and many people do not. If a woman feels hesitant or guilty about her sexual activity, she may be afraid that planning ahead to the extent of providing herself with contraception and using it will look calculating and make the activity less excusable. In this case, her failure to protect herself springs not so much from her feelings about pregnancy as from her feelings about sex. It can be a very hard thing to accept yourself as a sexually active person when society tells you that you are too young or too old, or that you shouldn't have sex with this one or that one because you are married or because you are not. Yet if you become pregnant, it is primarily you, not society, who must cope with the consequences.

Some women do not use contraception because they believe they are infertile. They may have been mistakenly told so, or they just think so. Often women become pregnant during menopause. Sometimes, if they resent the approaching loss of their fertility, they abandon contraception as an act of defiance. Sometimes they just don't know if they can safely stop taking precautions or not, and they don't like to ask because they are afraid an active sex life isn't appropriate at their age. (Though for many women, the completion of menopause actually marks the beginning of the first really enjoyable sex life they have ever had, because they are finally free of the fear of pregnancy.)

A lot of young women jump to the conclusion they are infertile for no clear reason. They just feel so inadequate, so bad about themselves, that they somehow come to believe that they can't conceive. They deliber-

ately use no contraceptives, partly because they are convinced it is unnecessary and partly because they would
like to be pregnant to prove they can do something
right. Some very young girls who have begun their sex
lives before they could in fact conceive—who therefore
have gone month after month without becoming pregnant—think this proves they are sterile. They may even
feel pressured to *try* to become pregnant to make sure
they can do it.

Thus the achievement of pregnancy may be im-
mensely satisfying, yet have nothing to do with wanting
a child. And the experience of becoming pregnant may
be repeated again and again. A woman may fear that,
even though she wasn't sterile before, she is now—as a
kind of punishment for having had an abortion or an
out-of-wedlock child.

The woman who has deliberately become pregnant,
or who has deliberately done nothing to prevent pregnancy although she does not want a child, obviously has
an immediate problem of deciding whether or not to
continue the pregnancy. But making that decision will
not necessarily solve the long-range problems that led
her to become pregnant in the first place.

Professional counseling can help. Confronting your
own conflicting emotions is difficult and complicated,
and the process can be made a lot easier by the partici-
pation of an objective and sympathetic listener.

A counselor can only help you to know yourself; your
final decision must still be your own. But there is one
important thing a counselor can do for you, if you feel
troubled, guilty, inadequate, or angry toward yourself
—and that is to help you find some source of strength
in your own life. A woman who feels that she is bad or
useless may believe that she has no one to count on or

turn to, that others feel about her as she feels about herself. It is hard to love others when you don't love yourself, and hard to trust others when you don't trust yourself.

On the other hand, you don't have to feel that professional counseling is indispensable. Often the greatest help of all to a woman who feels buffaloed, who is convinced she can't cope—is to cope.

It is a well-known maxim that when people want something done, they ask the busiest person around. The more you do for yourself the more you find you can do; the more you do nothing, the more you feel you are useless and *can* do nothing. In a period of crisis such as unplanned pregnancy many women find that they have strength they didn't know was there—that they have friends who love and trust them more than they knew. Life can push you and push you just so far; then, when you are up against the wall, you turn and fight.

Sometimes, if a woman has been told all her life that sex is bad and evil, she discovers, looking within herself, that she has come to feel *she* is bad and evil because she is a sexual person. She may have had sex deliberately to find out if it is *really* so evil—to see if lightning will strike her, or if she will be drastically marked or changed. If she then becomes pregnant, she may feel her worst fears were true—that she is being punished, perhaps that she deserves to suffer. She has to sort out her feelings of guilt and fear, to try to learn if they relate to her feelings about sex, or her feelings about pregnancy. She will then be better able to decide whether she is Being Punished or whether she is, in fact, punishing herself—and what course of action now is going to help her most to live with herself and her sense of her sexual nature.

It is also possible for some women to be pressured into having sex even though they don't really want to. Men tell them they are frigid if they don't Do It, other women tell them they haven't made it till they've Done It, books and magazines tell them that the really sensuous and liberated female covers herself with whipped cream every night and balls till the sun comes up. These are powerful pressures, and the woman who has given in to them may feel particularly angry with herself for not holding to her conviction that the decision *not* to have sex is as valid, mature, and liberated as the decision to have it. But again, before you can really decide how to handle the resulting pregnancy, you have to decide whether you are Being Punished, or whether you are just angry at yourself.

Some women have sex and become pregnant without really wanting either the sex or the pregnancy, but because their life situation forces them to make some dramatic statement about themselves. Sometimes, if a woman has domineering parents, or parents who demand so much of her that she feels she has no life of her own, she will become pregnant as a sort of Emancipation Proclamation—a way of saying, "I am an adult. My life is mine, my body is mine, and no one else can control it." Or the pregnancy is a way of getting the attention of parents—of saying, "I am important, I am capable of significant actions with lasting consequences, and I cannot be brushed aside." Whichever the reason —whether you have become pregnant to get your parents off your back or to make them face you as an adult —you now have to decide if the fact of pregnancy is enough of a statement, or if you also need and want to have a child. A woman in this position is likely to find herself under particularly strong pressure from her family to do what is in their best interest—to have an abortion if her condition embarrasses them, or to have a child. Under those circumstances, you will need to hold especially firm to your right to decide for yourself what is best for you.

If you are married, that also is apt to make you more vulnerable to pressure from outside sources. A married woman may be pressured by her husband to have sex though she fears the pregnancy that may result, pressured not to use contraceptives, pressured to have more and more children. She may even believe in her husband's right to make such decisions about the course of her life and the use of her body. If so, her response to an unwanted pregnancy will be that much more tormenting.

If she has no children and doesn't want any, she may be subjected to all sorts of threats and accusations. She may be called "selfish," "unnatural," or "unwomanly" —she may even come to believe such things about herself, and still wish to end her pregnancy. If she does have children, she may be told or she may feel herself that wanting an abortion means that she doesn't love the children she has. In her heart she probably knows this isn't true; she sees that loving one husband doesn't make her want three more husbands. But the very thought makes her feel guilty; and when from time to time she feels the natural resentment and irritation against her children that every parent occasionally feels, she takes that, too, as a sign that she is an unnatural mother.

If you are really in conflict with yourself about your right to control what happens to you, your conflict is bound to touch every aspect of your marriage, your attitude toward your husband and children, your feelings about yourself as a wife and a woman. One paragraph cannot illuminate it; your present crisis cannot resolve it.

But you certainly should know that the decision to bear a child or not is yours. You do not need your husband's consent to have an abortion, any more than any woman needs a man's consent to continue a pregnancy.

If you are considering going on with your pregnancy, it is important to take into account, as well as you can, your present and future emotional resources and, to some extent, financial ones.

A married woman, if she already has several children, needs to decide whether she has the physical and emotional energy to take on another child without impairing her ability to give and respond to the family she has. Realistically, she may also have to think whether the economic cost is something the family can deal with.

An unmarried woman who plans to have and raise an unplanned child needs to consider her resources, and to think about them in relation to the social pressures and hardships that are probably in store for her. Many women decide ultimately that they want to have the experience of motherhood even though they can't or don't want to marry—more and more of them, as the stigma of the Unwed Mother begins to fade in certain segments of society. On the other hand, raising a child alone is no easy matter, as many single, widowed, or divorced parents can attest; and if a woman is counting on the emotional and financial support of her friends, lover, or family, she had better be pretty sure they will be willing and able to stand by her when she needs them.

Recently, there have been several cases of glamorous and prominent women—Vanessa Redgrave and Mia Farrow, to name two—who have had highly publicized out-of-wedlock pregnancies. Thereupon a substantial number of other women decided that what was good enough for movie stars was good enough for them, and also opted to continue their pregnancies and to keep their children. When it turned out that unwed parenthood was considerably more difficult for those who are not wealthy and beautiful, and whose handsome and famous lovers do not marry them immediately after the delivery of twins, many of them turned to their mothers for help in raising their children, only to find that their mothers were unable or unwilling to become parents again. The result was that adoption agencies reported an unusually high number of one-year-old children being suddenly placed for adoption—a tragedy, because an older child has a smaller chance of being adopted than an infant.

All of which is by way of saying that if you want to have and keep a child out of wedlock, things are by no means as tough as they used to be. But if you are depending on help from someone else, you certainly owe it to yourself and to that person to talk it over and reach a firm understanding in advance.

Who's the One to Talk To?

Except in a case where your decision is directly dependent on what someone else may or may not do—as when you expect the help of a parent or friend in raising a child—it is difficult to know whom you should tell about your dilemma.

Obviously, you need someone who will support you, trust you, and believe in you. Equally obviously, it should also be someone who will not try to influence you one way or the other; you are under quite enough pressure from your own emotions. To seek out someone who is sure to be angry or hurt or upset may just be a way of hurting yourself. Parents may be so taken up with what your pregnancy means to them that they lose sight of what it means to *you*. A husband or lover can be even more confused and confusing. A man can have just as painful and conflicting emotions about a pregnancy in which he is involved as a woman; and he, too, may be more concerned with what is best for him than with what is best for you. The terrible truth is that every situation is different. It can turn out that the people who are closest to you and love you most are the least able to help you at this time, or that your crisis will bring out the best in them. Only you—if anyone—can predict which it will be.

But one thing is sure. Sooner or later you will probably have to tell *somebody*—either because you need money, or because you just need to talk to someone who knows you. And somebody in your life *should* know of your decision, whatever it is, because you are facing a period of heavy emotional and physical strain and there ought to be someone to help or take over for you should the need arise. That's a gloomy way to look at it, but there's no point in pretending that emergencies never come up when you know they do. The person you tell may be someone very close to you, but it doesn't have to be—after all, no matter how close he or she is, you'll still be the only one actually going through this experience. For some people the best help is a casual friend or a not-so-close relation like an aunt or cousin—people who care, who like you and want to help, but whose egos are not so involved that their self-interest conflicts with yours.

Maybe there is literally no one you feel you can confide in who will not make things more difficult for you; yet you want to talk out your anxieties. In that case, Planned Parenthood or the Clergy Consultation Service will be glad to help; or you can try calling a hospital family planning clinic, the Health Department or a local family agency, and asking to see a professional social worker who can help you to sort out your feelings. A professional social worker, by the way, is not just any person who makes a living nosing into other people's business. He or she has earned a specific graduate degree, a Master's degree in Social Work, and has had specific experience in what might be called informed listening.

Possibly you are a very private person who prefers to go your own way and to do it completely alone. Even so, it will be a good idea at least to let some professional person somewhere know that you *are* acting on your own. An abortion facility is apt to have social workers and trained counselors, as do adoption agencies and Birthright organizations whom you might contact for advice and assistance if you are going to go through with the pregnancy. You may not need or want help in making up your mind. But once you have made your decision, help in carrying it out is almost indispensable, and the above organizations will know better what kinds to offer if they are aware you have no one to lean on but yourself.

When Your Mind Is Made Up

If your decision is abortion, either Planned Parenthood or the Clergy Consultation Service will be able to tell you where to go and how to proceed. Be sure to report accurately the date of your last menstrual period and how many weeks pregnant the doctor said you were when you had the pregnancy diagnosed. This is particularly important if you are going to have to travel any distance to get the abortion, and if they are going to set up the appointment for you; they need to avoid sending you off too early and must also be sure you're not too far along to be accepted at a particular clinic or hospital.

If your decision is to continue your pregnancy, you can also call Planned Parenthood to find out where to get prenatal care and/or help in arranging an adoption. A Birthright or a Lifeline office in your area is another possibility for information, counseling, referral, and some financial aid. If you don't find either listed in your phone book, call the local Catholic Charities office for the number of the office nearest you. If you prefer, call the Jewish Community Service for the same services. These organizations are administered and funded by Catholic and Jewish organizations, respectively, but all serve women of any faith.

You can also get in touch with any adoption agency for counseling, prenatal care, and financial aid. This in no way commits you to putting the child up for adoption. You make no firm decision until after the baby is born, and until the social worker assigned you by the agency is sure that you are calm and positive about what you really want.

If you have decided to go through with the pregnancy and find you are going to need total financial support—

because you're simply on your own, or because you want to go to a shelter for unwed mothers during the period after the pregnancy becomes obvious—you can get help from the State or local Department of Social Services, Public Assistance or Welfare. You can call them yourself, or another agency will make the call for you.

3

The Modern
Clinic Abortion

If you have decided on an abortion and are less than twelve weeks pregnant, the surgical procedure ahead of you is relatively simple. If you are in good health, it is about the same kind of physical shock to your system as having a wisdom tooth out—which is to say, having a wisdom tooth extracted is probably a slightly bigger deal than you thought, and abortion not so big.

There is no reason why a procedure that goes according to routine couldn't be performed in a doctor's office —except that for one woman in a hundred it does not go routinely, and if this happens, certain emergency facilities had better be immediately available. Ideally, all abortions—the 99 routine procedures as well as the one that goes sour—ought to be performed in hospitals, or in clinics that either have the needed emergency equipment on their own premises or can quickly transport the patient to a nearby hospital. This is the way it was done in New York City after legalization, and helps account for the excellent safety record there.

A regular or general hospital obviously has the most complete emergency setup, but the doctor's bill, the anesthetist's bill, and the bill for an overnight stay can run into money. Hospital insurance rarely covers more than $100 of the total fee, which can run as high as $600 for even a routine procedure. The average is from $200 to $300. Certainly, this cost is well worth it to any patient with a special medical condition that might cause problems, but when they have a choice most women prefer an outpatient procedure—an arrangement that allows them to go home the same day as the abortion, usually after about three hours.

Inexpensive outpatient procedures are done by some hospitals. Much more commonly they are done in special "free-standing" clinics, which may provide abortion only or an assortment of other family planning services as well. These clinics have doctors and nurses and all the necessary equipment for routine procedures. Some have arrangements with a nearby "back-up" hospital, which insures that in case of emergency a patient will be admitted to the hospital at once and have available to her all its resources for treatment—whatever she needs. A few may even keep an ambulance at the clinic door.

Some free-standing abortion clinics are run by nonprofit organizations; some are frankly in business to make money. All charge a fee, which can range from $100 to $250 for an outpatient procedure. At nonprofit clinics, the fee is adjustable and no woman is ever denied an abortion for lack of money. But she is asked to pay as much of the fee as she honestly can; this is essential if they are to stay in operation.

Sometimes patients at the profit-making (proprietary) clinics feel that the staff is more concerned with the fee than with their well-being. Technically, the quality of medical care at the commercial clinics is probably as good as anywhere else—botched abortions are bad for business. But it is true that the psychological atmosphere can be cold and staff attitudes insensitive. Of course, nurses and counselors can feel harried or impatient anywhere, so it is possible to have an unpleasant experience at any kind of facility, regardless of its auspices—and equally possible that you will be treated with utmost sensitivity anywhere.

One distinction, though, of nonprofit clinics is that they believe that abortion should be offered in a context of a whole range of services related to running one's own reproductive life. Thus the abortion patient isn't isolated; neither is she thrown in with women having full-term deliveries as she may be in a hospital. They also are run pretty much alike, with a similar objective —to try to be a kind of medical establishment that serves patients as people, not numbers, and sees each of them as a whole person, not just a uterus or a pocketbook.

The description of a typical outpatient abortion experience given here is based on the procedures followed at one of these clinics—Planned Parenthood of New York City's 22nd Street Center in Manhattan. They are essentially what you will find at other nonprofit clinics, in New York City or elsewhere, though naturally every clinic will do things in its own way, and no one patient's experience is exactly like anyone else's, for people and circumstances vary from day to day.

But what follows are certainly the basics of almost any legal early abortion—what questions are asked you and why, what tests are done and why, and what the actual abortion is like. It may be more than you want to know. We have tried to include as much information as possible, because an abortion patient has enough on her mind without being troubled by misconceptions about what is being done and why it is being done.

On the other hand, you may have questions that won't be answered here. If so, be assured that wherever you go for your abortion you will be welcome to ask about anything that is not clear to you. (In fact, it is a good idea to jot them down in advance.) Many patients feel shy or embarrassed about asking questions, but believe this: *no* question is too simple or silly to ask when it concerns your health or peace of mind. Understanding what is happening to you is good for your head, and it is good medicine. Remember that nobody is doing you a favor by providing you with an abortion. You have a right to service that is not only medically excellent, but as comfortable as possible psychologically.

Making an Appointment

When you first telephone the clinic, you simply say you want an abortion. The interviewer who takes your call then asks you a series of questions.

If you aren't expecting them, it can feel as if you are being cross-examined. When you're nervous and jumpy, it feels like an attack if someone as much as asks how old you are. But all information is confidential, and each question is asked for a specific purpose—either to help them prepare your medical charts before you arrive for the abortion, or to discover at once if there is some reason why you should not have an outpatient procedure. (If there is, you will be told precisely where and whom to call to arrange an in-hospital abortion.)

At the outset you will be asked your name, and whether you have ever been a patient at any Planned Parenthood Center before (so they can locate their medical records of you, if any).

Then they will want to know the first day of your last menstrual period (LMP), and whether you have had your pregnancy confirmed by a doctor. If you have not, they will probably suggest that you have a pregnancy test at the Center; and if you are pregnant, the cost of the test will be included in the overall price of the abortion. If you live at some distance, they may recommend that you have the test done in your local community. If you have had a doctor's examination, they will need to know how many weeks pregnant the doctor found you to be.

You will then be asked the following questions about your medical history: Have you ever been treated for epilepsy? Are you a diabetic under treatment? Have you had an asthma attack in the last year? Are you allergic to novocaine? Have you been hospitalized for a nervous breakdown or other mental illness? Have you had any Caesarean sections? Are you under treatment for high blood pressure or heart disease? Have you had any recent serious illnesses or operations?

If the answer to any of these questions is yes, it does *not* mean that you cannot have an abortion. A yes to certain questions simply alerts the clinic doctor to things he should bear in mind in treating you at the clinic. A yes to others will only mean that you will be advised to go into a hospital with complete emergency facilities on the premises. And if you *are* advised to go to a hospital, that doesn't mean anyone actually expects you to have any trouble—just that if by some chance an emergency does come up, the clinic will not have the equipment to handle it but the hospital will.

You will be asked your age. If you are under seventeen, you will be asked if you have parental consent to have an abortion. If you do not, your appointment card will be marked so that a social worker will be ready to talk to you when you arrive—not to interrogate you and not to refuse you service, just to be sure you are firm about wanting an abortion. By the same token, when a minor is being pressured by parents or friends to have an abortion she doesn't want, the social worker can support her in her decision to continue the pregnancy. Also, if you wish you could share your decision with your parents but you are worried about their reaction, you can ask the social worker to talk to them—at the clinic or over the phone, even long distance. She won't *tell* them for you, but she may be able to explain your feelings to them more effectively than you can.

A minor is, of course, not the only one who can ask for and get this kind of help. If a patient of any age feels unsure about what she wants to do, she can ask to see a social worker when she arrives at the clinic. You should feel absolutely free to change your mind at any time; *no one* will be in the least disconcerted if you do, even at the very last minute.

You will be told the cost of the complete abortion service. At the 22nd Street Center this is on a sliding scale; the maximum is currently $145. This includes the cost of a pregnancy urine test, blood tests, Rhogam if

you need it to prevent Rh problems with future pregnancies, the abortion itself, contraceptive service if you
want it, and a postoperative checkup at the clinic. (At
other clinics, when you make an appointment be sure
to ask what the fee includes. Sometimes you have to pay
extra for the lab tests or Rhogam, and the Rhogam
charge alone can run as much as $80.) If you have
Medicaid, the abortion may be covered, depending on
what state you live in. Otherwise you will be asked to
bring a certified check, money order, travelers checks,
or BankAmericard with you to the clinic. If you cannot
possibly get together the money for the full fee before
your appointment, discuss it with the interviewer.

You will be told that the anesthetic used at the Center
is local—you will be awake during the abortion. If you
prefer an anesthetic that will put you to sleep, or if you
are allergic to the kind of anesthetic used at the clinic,
you will be referred to a hospital or another clinic. You
will be asked to eat or drink nothing, starting eight
hours before the time of the appointment. This is just
in case you should, by any mischance, need emergency
treatment—because it would then be essential that you
have nothing in your stomach or system that might
prevent the hospital from diagnosing and treating you
at once. (Some people think they are asked not to eat
because of the pregnancy test, and that they can eat
something after they give a urine sample. No such luck.)

Finally, you will be told to plan on being in the clinic
a total of five or six hours. The maximum time should
be allowed for when you arrange for child care while
you are gone, or when making travel plans for going
home; so if the only plane you can take back leaves at
one in the afternoon, better raise the point with the
interviewer now. You will also be asked not to bring any

cash or valuables with you, and to provide yourself with a sanitary belt for the sanitary napkin you will be wearing home. You will be urged to have a friend accompany you—or at least to have someone to go home with you. If you absolutely can't, they may suggest that you bring cab fare, so that you won't have to stand in the subway all the way back to Brooklyn. If at all possible, you should plan to take it easy and pamper yourself for the rest of the day on which you have the abortion, though you will probably feel fine. By the following day you should be able to resume normal activities. Specific instructions will be given before you leave the clinic.

The chances are you will be given an appointment for an abortion within three days or so of your call. If you are close to the 12th-week-of-pregnancy cutoff point, you may be taken even sooner. On the other hand, if you are in your sixth week, the clinic may ask you to wait a week or possibly two, especially if it is your first pregnancy. This is because your cervix (the round, muscular neck of the uterus) is very firm and tight if it has never been stretched by childbirth. By the seventh or eighth week of pregnancy it begins to stretch and soften of its own accord; before then, trying to dilate it might mean running an unnecessary risk. If for some very pressing reason you feel you can't wait, the clinic may agree to serve you early; but if the circumstances aren't compelling, you are probably better off sitting out the extra time.

The Day of the Abortion

Your appointment will be for eight, nine, or ten o'-clock in the morning—early, so you don't have to starve all day long. Anywhere from five to fifteen other women will have appointments at the same time as you. The receptionist will greet you, record your arrival, and give you a form to fill out.

The information on the form—as well as all information you are asked for throughout the day—is *absolutely* confidential. Primarily, the purpose of the facts you provide is to help the clinic to serve you better; partly, it is to enable the clinic and the Health Department to keep the kind of records necessary to assess and improve health procedures in the future.

The waiting room at the Center is large and comfortable, since anyone who accompanies you is going to be spending several hours there. Adjoining it is a small playroom with toys and a blackboard if you are bringing your children. There is no full-time play-person, though, so if you do bring children it will be best if an adult comes with you to help keep them occupied. If this is not possible, the staff will do their best to help out whenever they have a minute free.

The name of your companion or any person who is coming later to go home with you will be recorded, and if anyone is going to call in to check on you during the day you should also leave his or her name at the desk. No one else will be told that you are there or given any information about you. You will be called by your first name throughout the day—not in the familiar way that salesladies call you "dear," but in order to keep the atmosphere informal and to preserve your anonymity.

When everyone scheduled at the same time as you has arrived and filled in an information sheet, the group of you are taken to the patient waiting areas. Your group will be accompanied throughout the day by three to six members of the clinic staff—nurses, social workers, or other trained people specializing in work with abortion patients. They will shepherd you from one part of the clinic to another, collect some necessary data, fill in your forms, and take a few simple tests; but above all, they are supposed to be there to help you.

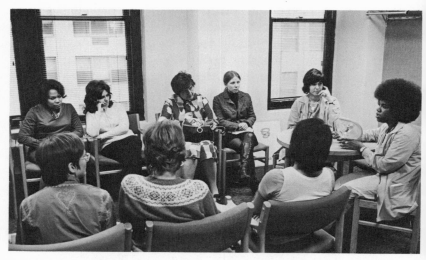

Before having their abortions, patients meet in a group with staff members of Planned Parenthood of New York City's 22nd Street Center to learn about the procedure and to have their questions answered.

They will begin your day with a group orientation session. This gives them a chance to answer your questions and tell you what will be happening. It also gives you a chance to size *them* up—to see by the way they listen and talk that they want to help and that they have no desire to judge. At the same time, another staff person will be in the front waiting room explaining the day's procedures to the assorted husbands, lovers, friends, and parents who have come with the patients.

In your group session, one of the staff explains the purpose of the laboratory and medical tests you will have, and with the help of a transparent plastic model of your vital parts, she describes the vacuum aspiration procedure. She informs you that in addition to the physician, a nurse will be with you throughout the procedure and, in some cases, a counselor as well. Some patients find these meetings interesting and reassuring, some find them boring or disturbing. They are offered to everybody, so that each patient can make her own choice—to participate or not. If your choice is not to participate, you can plug your ears or read a book; you are in a medical facility, not a girl scout camp.

The formal part of the orientation meeting ends with a discussion of some forms of contraception. After that, there is time for you to ask questions.

Oddly enough, no matter what terror, anger, or regret they may have been feeling the night before, the first thing on most people's minds the day of the abortion is *hunger*. Almost everyone asks when they can eat and what they will have. The answer is you can eat half an hour after you get to the recovery room, and you will have your choice of a dazzling array of lovely cinnamon toast, four kinds of lovely soup, and lovely tea or coffee.

The next most-asked question is about the shot of anesthetic: when is it given, where is it given, and how much does it hurt. To this, the reply is that the anesthetic is given after the doctor finishes his examination of your uterus. The needle goes up the vagina into the cervix, not through the abdomen. And since the cervix is not especially sensitive, the shot just feels like a hard pinch, and you will have a couple of them, one on either side of the cervix.

Some women ask what becomes of the tissue that is removed during the abortion. It is sent to a laboratory for analysis, as is all tissue removed during any surgical procedure. In this case, the lab is checking to be sure fetal material is included. If it were not, it might mean that the abortion was incomplete, or that the fetal material was in the Fallopian tube instead of in the uterus—a rare but quite dangerous occurrence which would have to be corrected surgically. Or the woman was not pregnant at the time of the abortion; and in that case, it would be important to find out at once what *was* happening in her uterus that made her appear to be pregnant.

Some women want to know if they have to see the material that has been removed. The answer to that is no, though you probably can if you want to; you can ask the doctor when you see him or her.

Some ask if you can tell if it would have been a boy or a girl. You can't tell, at this point; sex differentiation doesn't become visible until about the thirteenth week of pregnancy.

A good many women ask when they should expect to menstruate again. They are told that the abortion counts as the first day of a menstrual period, and the next period will arrive four to six weeks later.

Some women wonder if the abortion will affect their fertility. Almost certainly, it will not. Within about two weeks of an abortion, the vast majority of women are ovulating and as fertile as ever. If a serious infection were to set in after the abortion—and *if* the infection were to go untreated—then there might be some risk of sterility; or if the cervix were to be damaged, a woman might be more likely to miscarry late in a future pregnancy. But when an early abortion is done under proper conditions, the odds are greatly against either of these events occurring. There is some indication that *repeated* abortions may eventually cause infertility—but nobody knows for sure why, or how many is too many.

When the orientation is over, the patients go in twos and threes to the lavatory to produce urine samples, then into the lab to give blood samples. The blood is taken by hypodermic needle from a vein in your arm and goes into a tube the size of a cigar; it fills about one and a half inches of the tube.

In the lab, the urine is tested for the hormone that indicates pregnancy; then it is broken down for general analysis just to make sure you have no mysterious infections and are generally healthy. The blood is tested for type (if you didn't know before what type you are, they will be happy to tell you) and for Rh factor.

Everybody is either Rh positive or Rh negative, and you probably know that the child of an Rh negative mother and an Rh positive father can be born with a serious disease—erythroblastosis. What you may not know is that when an Rh negative woman carries an Rh positive fetus, either birth or abortion can cause antibodies to build up in the woman's blood and these may, in turn, endanger the health of her future children. It is to prevent this—if the lab test indicates it is necessary —that you will be given a shot of Rhogam at the time of the abortion; Rhogam prevents the antibodies from forming in your blood.

The blood sample is also subjected to a hematocrit— to check iron levels, and again to establish that you are generally healthy.

Orientation and lab work may take from forty-five minutes to an hour, depending on how large your group is and how busy the clinic is. After the lab work you wait your turn for an individual interview. The wait may be a few minutes or as much as a half hour, and during this time you sit in the patient waiting area with the other women in your group.

A good deal of comfort and information is exchanged among patients at this point. Sometimes it helps you to feel better about yourself just to see that so many other normal, intelligent individuals are in exactly the same situation. Sometimes one woman will have had an abortion before, and she can be more reassuring than all the cheerful social workers in the world. But no one will be surprised if you don't feel like chatting, and if you expect to be feeling private, bring a book or magazine or some knitting. People are less apt to bother you if you seem to be busy; besides, it is good to have something to occupy you through all the sitting around, which is the most unpleasant part of the whole day. (Except, maybe, the hunger.)

The Personal Interview

As soon as possible, one of the clinic staff will call your name, and you will go with her to a consultation room for a private interview.

If you have any special complaints, fears, or questions, now is the time to bring them up. Your interviewer will try to give you whatever opening you need to talk about anything that is bothering you, and there is nothing you can ask or say that she hasn't heard before. But if you don't feel like talking, that's OK, too —the interview is for your benefit, not hers.

First, she will ask you a series of questions about your reproductive history. She will need to know what your

normal periods have been like since you began men-
struating, and about any previous pregnancies you may
have had. From your answers the doctor will know as
much as possible about your uterus when he or she
actually confronts it.

Next, she will take down your medical history—
much more detailed than the few items you were asked
about on the phone. Some of her questions will bear
only on your own past health; some will also apply to
health problems that run in your family, even if you
yourself haven't been affected.

Now, more than ever, it is important that you answer
these questions honestly and accurately. If you have a
health problem, you may be afraid you will be denied
an abortion if you tell the clinic anything about it, and
the temptation to conceal it is enormous. More than one
woman has felt she would rather run any risk than be
turned away after getting so far. But more than one has
lost the gamble. The rate of complications in early abortion has been very low in New York since the state law
was liberalized, but there have been some; and the complications that have arisen have stemmed, by and large,
from one of two causes. Either the abortion was attempted too early or too late; or the patient concealed
some vital aspect of her medical record, such as severe
asthma or a history of convulsions, so that when an
emergency arose, the clinic or hospital could not cope
with it quickly enough.

Next, the interviewer will take your pulse, blood pressure, and temperature, and give you a consent form to
sign. She will also ask you for an address or phone
number at which the clinic can reach you or leave a
message after the procedure, if they need to—say, if

your Pap smear or tissue analysis shows up something that should be checked. It needn't be your home address or phone, if you prefer not. They will respect your wishes unquestioningly; but in that case, the interviewer will ask for your home address and phone, too—solely for use in the event of a serious emergency.

Now that she has filled up all your medical records, the interviewer will ask you a few more questions, usually more personal than any that have gone before. This is to help both her and you to assess your state of mind. If you seem agitated, she will ask you a little about yourself and your feelings to see if together you can get at the source of your agitation and deal with it. If you are very calm she may probe a little, to discover if you really have nerves of steel or if you are secretly falling apart inside. She may ask you about your sexual activity, how you feel about your pregnancy, how you feel about the man involved or why you want an abortion. The point is not that she wants to know, but that she wants to be sure that you do. She may ask if you have been using birth control. If you say no, she may ask you why not; and when she does, no matter how she says it, it's going to sound like *"Oh yeah? Why not, YOU DUMBBELL?"*

She is aware of this and regrets it. But right now she feels she has to reach out to you as directly as she can, *not* because she wants to upset you, but because at this critical moment you are in a sensitive state—highly aware of your fertility, intensely mindful of its consequences—and she is trying to help you to make the moment count.

You may feel angry at being talked to in such a way, especially if you feel that in the course of decision-making you have already gotten your feelings together by yourself; but if you have done so completely, you are lucky. For many of us, our feelings about men, sex, pregnancy, and motherhood are so complicated that we don't really face them without being pushed, and we don't even realize we aren't facing them except at a moment of crisis like this.

There is also a specific practical reason for bringing up contraception at this point—before the abortion. As you know, any birth control method you choose is available to you as part of the whole abortion service. You have heard the various methods described during the orientation session, and you will hear them discussed in depth later in the recovery room. You need not have made up your mind yet which, if any, you want to use; but if you have—and if your choice is the Pill or the IUD—then it can save you a delay in getting protection if you say so now. The doctor can insert the IUD in your uterus immediately after the abortion while the cervix is still dilated—or if you want pills, his examination of you will be done with that in mind, and if there are no contraindications, you can start your first package of pills at once. The alternative in both cases is to wait an entire month or more—till your period comes, and for some women this would be an inconvenience if not a hardship.

The final thing the interviewer will need to talk over with you is the matter of the fee, which—since it is on a sliding scale—may mean some questions about your financial setup. If you have brought the agreed-upon amount with you, she will note that on your fee slip. If not, you can discuss arrangements for paying off the balance later.

The Examination and the Abortion

After your interview, you may have another brief wait or you may be taken immediately to a small dressing room off the procedure room. Here you will be asked to remove all your clothes, which will be put in a shopping bag with your name on it and kept all together for you until after the abortion.

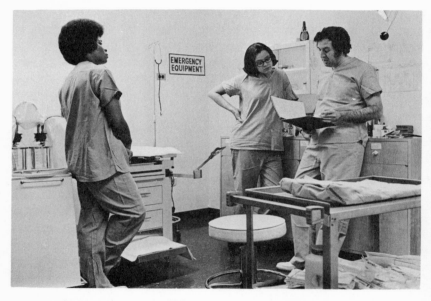

An operating room of Planned Parenthood of New York City's 22nd Street Center. From left to right, the nurse, counselor, and physician review the medical record of their next abortion patient. At far left is the vacuum aspirator; behind the nurse is the gynecological table; on the tray in the foreground is the package of sterile instruments.

You then put on a hospital gown (the kind that flops open in the back) and go into the procedure room. This is somewhat larger than the examining room of a doctor's office, with a stand for sterile instruments, lights, and a gynecological table. With you will be a doctor, a nurse, and, if possible, the same staff worker who just interviewed you.

The doctor will listen to your heart and lungs and check your breasts for any lumps that shouldn't be there; then you will lie on the table with your hips at the end and your feet in metal stirrups, as you did for your pelvic exam when your pregnancy was diagnosed. If anything happens that you don't understand, you can ask about it.

Instruments used in performing an early abortion. From top: a sponge stick for washing the vagina; a tenaculum, for grasping the cervix; a uterine probe; a cervical dilator; a vacuum curette, to be attached to the end of the aspirator tube; a placental tissue forceps, used to remove any tissue not easily removed by the aspirator; and a regular spoon-shaped curette. At the upper right hand corner is a solution cup for antiseptic liquid; below it is a vaginal speculum, lying on gauze sponges. For an actual abortion, the tray also contains several cervical dilators of different widths, and additional curettes.

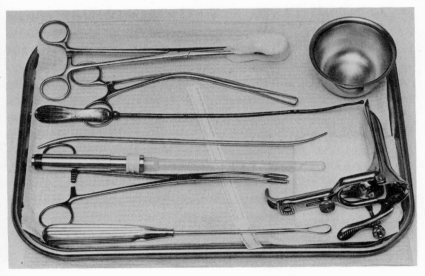

First, the doctor will perform another pelvic examination, checking the uterus to reconfirm that you are not too early, or, more importantly, too late, and to help him know what to expect when he begins the abortion. Since this is probably your second thorough pelvic examination in a very short time, it may seem excessive. Yet the doctor really does need to check you himself, even though you may have a perfectly good letter with you confirming that you are healthy and eight weeks pregnant. For one thing, doctors' opinions differ; and even more importantly, uteri differ—they come in different shapes and different positions, and he must familiarize himself with yours. If all is well, the abortion will now begin.

To start with, the doctor sprays your vagina with a cold disinfectant solution. He puts the speculum in place to hold the walls of the vagina open, and again takes a Pap smear from the cervix.

Next, he grasps the cervix with a tenaculum—a metal instrument shaped like a pair of scissors, except that it has clamps at the tip instead of blades. It serves to hold the uterus steady; ordinarily it floats and bobbles around a bit inside you.

You may feel a pinch when the tenaculum takes hold, but it is important that you lie perfectly still; you now have instruments inside you, and any jerk or sudden movement could cause you to injure yourself. If you feel tense, you can talk or be talked to.

Try to relax as much as possible. It will make you feel better and it will actually decrease physical discomfort. Just let your lower body go limp and keep your legs spread wide, and if you want to clench anything, clench your teeth.

Now come the shots, one on either side of the cervix

—more if necessary. The anesthetic numbs the cervix and the uterus; though you probably won't be aware of much numbness, since you don't ordinarily get many messages from these organs anyway. It takes two minutes or less for the anesthetic to take effect.

After exploring the uterus a little with a probe, the doctor begins to dilate the cervix. To do this he uses metal instruments called dilators which slide into the cervical opening, making it spread. The thinnest dilator, about as big around as a match stick, is slipped in and removed; it is replaced with a fatter one and then a fatter one until the opening in the cervix is about as big around as a fountain pen or larger.

This is the only part of the procedure that can cause much discomfort. The cervix is a muscle, and when muscles expand and contract you sometimes feel cramps. If you usually get cramps during your period, you will probably get them now; if you usually do not, you may not be bothered at all. You can ease things by breathing deeply—in through your nose and out through your mouth, as long as you feel the cramps. (If you haven't been shown how already, you will be now.) This helps you to relax, relieves whatever pressure on your lower organs has been caused by your tense diaphragm, and rushes oxygen to the cramped muscles.

When the cervix is dilated you are ready for the aspirator. The machine itself consists of a small enclosed vacuum motor with two bottles on top. The bottles are attached to a long hollow tube, the end of which is fitted with a blunt-tipped vacuum curette. Curettes are about six inches long and have different-sized openings at the tip—the right size for you will depend on how pregnant you are.

The doctor inserts the vacuum curette into the uterus

through the dilated cervical opening and turns on the motor. It makes a low, whirring-motor sound; someone will warn you when it is coming. Then the contents of the uterus are gently sucked out through the tube. You will feel this, not as pain, but as a strange pulling sensation inside of you. It takes a very short time, usually from one to five minutes.

When it is over, the motor is turned off, and the doctor removes the vacuum curette. He replaces it with a regular, spoon-shaped curette, which he glides around the inside of the uterus. He is checking to be sure everything is out, and listening for a certain sound—a hollow uterus makes a sound something like sandpaper being rubbed by your hand. (Don't expect to be able to hear it yourself.) If you are having an IUD put in, it will be inserted as soon as the doctor finishes the curettage.

Then the speculum and the tenaculum are removed, and the nurse cleans you up a bit, swabbing off excess disinfectant and so on. You will be bleeding a little—about as much as you do when you have your period—so you will be given a sanitary pad to catch the flow. As soon as you are ready, you sit up and get down from the table. You are given a pair of natty little paper slippers, and escorted to the recovery room.

You may feel a little dizzy, shaky, or faint. Partly this is because your system has had a small shock; partly it is the aftereffect of the anesthetic. And partly it is because by this time, you are really ravenously hungry.

Recovery

The Center has a single big recovery room with hospital beds in one area, and lots of big lounge chairs in the other.

For the first twenty minutes or so you lie in bed. A nurse records the time of your arrival in Recovery, and checks your vital signs—blood pressure, pulse, breathing, and so on. As you lie in bed, any cramping you still feel will subside. You may feel a little nausea, from emotional strain and hunger. Most people feel surprisingly good, happy and relieved. Some feel sad, especially if they wanted and didn't want the pregnancy in equal measure. You may feel like crying, or somebody in the room with you may be crying—from sadness or from relief or a combination of the two.

One Center staff member recalls being with an unmarried woman whose child was waiting for her in the reception room. After the abortion the woman began to cry, and the staff worker asked her if she could help— if the abortion had made her feel depressed. The woman said that it had and it hadn't—that she was really crying because she was thinking how different her life would have been if an abortion had been available to her ten years ago.

While you are in bed, someone will come to talk to you about your postoperative checkup. If you want to come back to the clinic for it, an appointment will be made for you then and there. If you are going to go to your own doctor for the checkup, you will be urged to do so in about two weeks. You will be told not to douche or take tub baths (showers are fine), not to use tampons, and not to have sexual relations of any description during these two weeks. The idea is to avoid introducing anything into the vagina that might cause infection at this critical time—before a doctor has confirmed that the uterus is completely healed and back to its normal nonpregnant size. While you are lying down, you may be given an antibiotic to prevent infection and perhaps a drug such as ergotrate to help the uterus contract, especially if it was large or if there was a lot of bleeding. If you have picked a birth control method, you will be handed a sheet of instructions about its use.

After twenty minutes or a half hour, the nurse will check your vital signs again. You can then get up, dress, and go into the lounge-chair area to read, talk, or play scrabble, and at last be fed. After you have eaten, if you want to, you can go out to the reception room for a few minutes to talk to anyone waiting for you and show that you are all right.

Abortion patients relax in the lounge area of the recovery room at Planned Parenthood of New York City's 22nd Street Center.

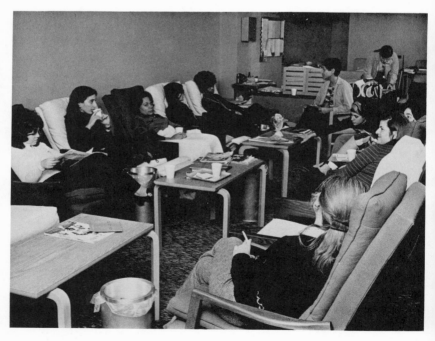

You will rest in one of the recovery room chairs for about two and a half hours, making a total of three that have elapsed since the abortion. This gives you time to pull yourself together and to be watched over and checked for any untoward symptoms. If you feel you have a compelling reason for leaving earlier, it is possible to sign yourself out; but you would have to sign a release form absolving the clinic of all responsibility for any complications that might arise, and it is really not a great idea.

While you are resting, there will be another detailed group discussion of contraceptives, at which point you may feel as if they are twisting your arm about the subject, but some patients aren't really ready to listen until now. Anyway, nobody can or wants to make you choose a method if you'd rather not, and you can read or sleep if you can't bear to hear about it again. The discussion usually ranges over a variety of subjects; men, sex, pregnancy—whatever the women feel like talking about. Meanwhile, the staff will be happy to jog back and forth with messages between you and anyone waiting for you.

Not infrequently, after the first hour or so in the recovery room, some of the women begin to feel restless and impatient. They suddenly want to know why they can't ask their husband or boyfriend to come in, why they can't have a steak instead of this toast-and-tea slop, and why they can't go home. More than likely they know perfectly well why—it is not fair to other patients, the clinic hasn't hired a chef yet, and medical supervision at this time is an important safeguard. But when you begin to feel yourself again after an abortion, one of the first reactions is often anger that it ever happened; and since you can't change that, you feel angry at the place where it happened instead. Cheer up—it is almost over.

The Exit Interview

When your recovery time is almost up, you will return to a private consultation room for an exit interview —a final opportunity to talk about how you feel, what the abortion has meant to you, and anything else concerning your physical or mental well-being that might be on your mind. You also have a last chance now to ask any questions you want to about your method of birth control, so that you and the interviewer can be sure you understand how it works and how to use it. At this time some women really feel like talking; some really feel like just getting out of there as soon as possible.

When you are ready to go, you will be reminded about not doing anything for two weeks that could introduce infection into the vagina, and about the importance of seeing a doctor as soon as possible after that time.

From the interview room, you go to the cashier's office to pay your bill, and from there you can go home. If you have no one accompanying you, someone will be glad to go downstairs with you and get you a cab if you want one.

Complications

Statistically the chance of any complication in a legal abortion done in the first twelve weeks of pregnancy is very low. But there are a few kinds of complications which possibly *could* occur during a surgical procedure of this kind.

The first is perforation of the uterus during the procedure—if the probe, the dilator, the aspirator tip, or the curette happens to poke through the wall of the uterus and damage internal organs beyond. The risk is greatest when the abortion is attempted while the cervix is too tight, or when a spot on the uterine wall has been weakened by previous surgery, such as a Caesarean section.

Perforations may turn out not to be serious at all— slight enough to heal themselves in time—or they may be very serious. At the moment they happen, though, there is no telling how much harm has been done; so when any perforation occurs in a free-standing clinic, the patient is transferred immediately to a stretcher kept just outside the procedure room, and she is rushed by ambulance to the back-up hospital whose emergency room is standing by and ready to treat her.

A second type of complication is hemorrhage, or heavy bleeding. During the procedure, it might be caused by perforation of the uterine wall, or it might take place inside the uterus at the place where the placenta is attached. If it begins after the abortion has been completed, some internal damage may have been done during the abortion that the doctor was not aware of; or it might mean that not all of the fetal material was removed.

If hemorrhaging begins while a patient is still in the clinic, she will be zoomed to the hospital where she can be treated with drugs and blood transfusions. If it begins later—and it could happen as much as a week later— she should call her doctor at once. She may be treated with drugs and, if necessary, a transfusion; she may also have to be readmitted to a hospital to have a D & C (dilation and curettage) to be sure the uterus is completely empty.

Hemorrhage should not be confused with normal bleeding after an abortion. Normal bleeding is about the same as your regular menstrual period; hemorrhaging is at least twice as much bleeding and possibly heavy clotting as well.

A third kind of complication is infection, caused by germs in the vagina or uterus before healing is complete. (This was always a great danger in illegal abortions, which were so often done with nonsterile instruments.) If germs are already present in the uterus before the abortion, infection might result from the patient's lowered resistance afterward. In the case of an incomplete abortion, tissue left in the uterus might breed infection. Or infection could occur if anything carrying germs enters a woman's vagina or uterus before her bleeding has stopped—the reason for the postoperative ban on swimming, tub baths, douches, tampons, vaginal sprays, and any kind of oral, manual, or genital intercourse.

Normally, this danger is past when two weeks have gone by; most women can then resume all their ordinary activities. But different women heal at different rates, and some will go on spotting for a couple of weeks more—and having to be careful of infection.

Finally, there is the chance of laceration of the cervix which, if it does occur, usually happens during dilation, and which could create a danger of late miscarriage in a future pregnancy. It happens occasionally, and it is one of the things the doctor checks for at the follow-up examination.

Post-Abortion Danger Signs

After the abortion, take things easy for the rest of the day. Next morning, if your bleeding is normal and you feel fine, do whatever you like; but it is best to avoid really strenuous activity for a few days. If you know in advance that you have something demanding scheduled for the next day—a gym class or your return to a physically arduous job—tell the doctor at the clinic before you leave. The chances are you will be able to proceed as usual. If not, you will be given a letter saying that you should be excused for the day—no reason has to be specified.

You may feel some residual weakness, soreness, or cramps on the day of the abortion. The soreness should go away quickly. If it becomes worse instead, or if you experience heavy bleeding, nausea, or vomiting, or if you run a fever of more than 100°, call the clinic or a doctor *at once*. You should also see a doctor if you have any unusual or bad-smelling discharge from the vagina, for this could indicate fetal tissue still in the uterus and possible infection.

In the days following the abortion, most women feel in surprisingly good spirits. You don't realize just how tense and nervous you were until the tension is gone. Also, it may be the first time in several weeks that you have really felt like eating, that you have slept well, and felt your old prepregnant energy.

But you may feel some depression and sadness, too —a sense of loss or regret that comes to some women after an abortion, just as it comes to some women after childbirth. When it happens after a normal delivery, it is called "post-partum blues." When it follows abortion, there is no cute name for it. Neither is there any magic cure. But there is a way to make it worse, and that is to deny it and bury it.

Before abortion was made legal, there were some doctors who opposed the procedure, not on medical or moral grounds, but because they believed it was emotionally dangerous to a woman. They felt they had grounds for their belief; they had seen many cases of women who experienced deep emotional or sexual problems because of unresolved feelings of fear, guilt, and sorrow stemming from an abortion.

Now, since abortion has been legalized, there is strong evidence that much of this difficulty was caused by the fact that the procedure was illegal. The natural distress the woman might have felt about the termination of the pregnancy itself was vastly magnified by the very real physical danger of the abortion procedure at that time, as well as by the humiliation associated with it and the knowledge that she was breaking a law. After the abortion, if she was still troubled by the experience, she was afraid to talk about it—again, because the procedure was illegal. Normal feelings that could have been dealt with were left to fester, or were perhaps suppressed for long periods, until at last they came back to her in the form of a sense of guilt and unworthiness she could no longer deal with; she didn't even remember herself exactly how she came to feel that way.

Knowing that you are legally free to make the choice of abortion helps to prevent a good deal of emotional confusion in the first place; and for a woman who is deeply and genuinely ambivalent about making a choice, there is professional counseling available all along the way. Afterward, talking about any depression you feel with a friend or relative who knows what you've been through, is enough, in most cases, to prevent your feelings from going deeper and coming back later to haunt you.

But if you should feel seriously depressed—and you should not expect to, because such a reaction is rare—by all means get in touch with a professional counselor, and the sooner the better. Call your local Planned Parenthood affiliate or a family planning clinic in your area, or the Health Department. Any of them should be able to put you in touch with a trained counselor or social worker who will know how to help you. In the case of emotional problems, an ounce of prevention is worth a ton of cure.

4

Late Abortions

The great majority of all legal abortions done in the last few years have been performed in the first twelve weeks of pregnancy. The procedure is certainly safest then; in New York City, for example, not a single death from an abortion done by the suction method has been recorded from July, 1971 through February, 1973 (the latest figures available at the time of this writing). And because many early abortions can be and are done on an outpatient basis, they are clearly less costly than late ones.

But around 20 percent of the women who have had abortions in New York have not been able to have early abortions, and for any of a number of reasons.

Some women may make up their minds in the first

month, yet delay getting the abortion because they don't have the money or the information to proceed. Some simply don't realize they are pregnant until late —especially if they are very young or approaching menopause, the ages at which cycles are often irregular. Other women may have particular difficulty in facing the fact that they are pregnant, or coming to grips with making a decision. Sometimes a pregnancy is wanted in the beginning; then something happens in a woman's life that radically changes her circumstances and her mind. Maybe the man involved has deserted her or died, or she has left him; perhaps financial or social pressures have made it impossible for her to continue a pregnancy she initially wanted. Or it may have just been discovered that the pregnancy is endangering the woman's health —or something has damaged the fetus, such as the woman's exposure to German measles or a drug known to cause birth defects.

As a pregnancy becomes more advanced, the decision-making process is often tougher, but the right to decide is still legally yours. And though the medical risk you run is higher—the chance of complications is about four times greater in a late abortion than in an early one, and the mortality rate about eight times higher—it is still a significantly lower risk, statistically, than childbirth carries.

If your last menstrual period began exactly twelve weeks ago, there is a possibility that even now an early abortion procedure can be performed, but the possibility is slim. Occasionally a woman who is twelve or even thirteen weeks from LMP has a uterus that is apparently less advanced—it looks like what is typical at the tenth or eleventh week. But things are just as apt to work the other way. Perhaps only eleven weeks have gone by since LMP; yet the uterus is so large that the vacuum method is out of the question and a D & C is highly likely to cause perforation or hemorrhage.

At this crucial stage of pregnancy, the doctor has to make the judgment, and what it is will depend on his reading of the condition of the uterus and his estimation of the possible risk. A few abortions are done by suction or D & C as late as the fourteenth week from LMP; but it is far more likely that you will be asked to wait out the entire so-called Interim Period—from the twelfth to the sixteenth weeks of your pregnancy. By that time, the uterus will have grown still larger—large enough for the doctor to use the method of abortion called salting out or, more formally, saline injection.

You will have to be hospitalized for a saline abortion, which accounts for its higher cost. The cost will probably be covered in full if you have Medicaid (this is the case in New York); but ordinary health insurance will, at best, only pay what it would for a full-term delivery —rarely more than $100. Some hospitals charge a fee based on patients' ability to pay; at others, the fee is from $300 or $350 up. Neither Planned Parenthood nor the Clergy Consultation Service refers patients to hospitals that charge substantially more than $350.

The Saline Procedure

The preoperative procedure for a late abortion is substantially the same as for an early one. You will have a thorough examination and you will be asked questions about your medical history. Blood and urine tests will be done to establish blood type and general health and check for any infections—especially kidney infections, for the kidneys are under strain during the saline abortion. Again, they will check for the Rh factor; and again, if you are negative, you will probably need a shot of Rhogam within 72 hours after the abortion to prevent problems with future pregnancies.

If everything is in order, you will walk to a treatment room—like a doctor's examining room, not an operating room. You will be asked to drink water before the procedure so that you won't become dehydrated when the salt in the saline solution is absorbed by your body. Then you will empty your bladder to prevent its being injured during the procedure.

When you are lying flat on the procedure table, the doctor will clean a patch on the middle of your abdomen with disinfectant, then numb the area with a local anesthetic such as Xylocaine (like Novocaine) injected with a fine needle.

When the anesthetic has taken effect, the doctor will reach for a hypodermic syringe with a needle about three and a half inches long. It looks grim, but it won't hurt, so if the sight of it upsets you, just look away. With it, the doctor is going to remove fluid from the amniotic sac around the fetus.

The doctor puts the needle through the numbed skin, the muscle beneath, and the wall of the uterus, into the amniotic sac. He may withdraw the fluid, or he may let it flow out by itself; altogether about two-thirds of a cup of fluid will be removed. The amount varies with the amount in the sac, which is close to a cup at sixteen weeks, a cup and a half at twenty weeks. The liquid may be cloudy or clear, or slightly pink with blood at the start. You can watch it or not. As the fluid is removed from the sac, the uterus begins to contract. Since these contractions might dislodge the rigid needle, some doctors replace the needle at this stage with a slender, flexible plastic tube.

When the right amount of fluid has been removed, it is replaced with an equal or smaller amount of salt-and-water solution, dripped into the sac through the same needle or tube. (They just change the bottle to which the tube is attached, so they don't have to be sticking anything else into you.) This infusion of the saline solution is done very slowly, so that if anything begins to go wrong it can be stopped at once; it may take as long as an hour. Most women feel no reaction to the solution, but if you should feel suddenly hot, or experience cramps or burning in your lower abdomen, say so. The procedure will stop, your head will be raised, and you will be given water to drink. When you feel better, the procedure can go on.

A saline abortion is done with a local anesthetic (rather than a general, that would put you to sleep) for two reasons. First, general anesthesia always carries with it some risks of its own, and imposes additional stress on the body; it is usually avoided in any procedure when local anesthetic will do as well. Second, it is particularly important in a saline abortion that the patient be awake so she can tell the doctor exactly how she feels. That way, if anything is wrong he can be alerted at once and can correct it. For instance, if the tip of the needle were to be touching the wall of the uterus instead of being in the sac, the woman would feel stinging pain as the salt entered the uterus. Or if the solution were to be injected into her blood stream, instead of the sac, she would begin to feel cold and sick or dizzy, with pain in her lower back where the kidneys are. You will be told to report such symptoms to the doctor quickly, for any of these occurrences could be dangerous if not corrected immediately.

When enough salt solution has been injected into the sac, the tube or needle is removed from your abdomen. You may feel a little crampy or nauseous, but you will probably just be thirsty. You will be told to drink lots of liquids and not eat anything salty. The chances are you won't be in much of a pretzels or popcorn mood.

At some point after this whole procedure is finished, the uterus begins to contract, as in labor, and push out the fetus and placenta. There is no way to predict the point at which the contractions will begin—it may be as soon as five hours after the infusion, or as late as two days. For most women, it comes between eight and 36 hours later. Some hospitals give an injection of hormone such as oxytocin to speed the onset of contractions. In those cases, the abortion is usually completed within twelve hours.

Most hospitals have the woman stay in bed in the hospital throughout the waiting period, but some allow her to go home with instructions to return when contractions begin. This enables the hospital to avoid having a bed taken up when nothing is happening, and it saves the patient the high cost of occupying it while she waits. She probably runs no great risk physically by going home, but it may be very hard on her emotionally unless she has a capable and informed companion with her; also, home certainly has to be near enough for her to get back to the hospital fast when labor begins. Some hospitals have saline abortion patients check into a nearby hotel with a trained attendant on call. But what is most likely—and what certainly is to be recommended—is that you will stay in the hospital for the entire time. Unfortunately, in all probability, you will be in its obstetrical section.

Sometime, perhaps, in the best of all possible futures, hospitals and clinics will have special facilities for the "surgical control of fertility"—areas exclusively reserved for patients having abortions and sterilizations. Most hospitals recognize the need for this, but because of the pressures of space and money, abortion patients are usually bedded down in the same area as full-term delivery patients. It is best to be aware of this because it can cause emotional strain—for you, and sometimes for the medical staff. It can be confusing and conflicting for some doctors or nurses to turn from the bedside of a patient who is trying to preserve a pregnancy to the bedside of another patient who is ending one. This by no means excuses the harsh and insensitive treatment an abortion patient can encounter, but you may find it easier to deal with if you are prepared for it.

When your uterus begins to contract, you will recognize the sensations as being like labor pains, if you have had a child before; or they may seem to you like an extreme form of the cramps that accompany your period. The uterus hardens when it contracts—then it relaxes. You can probably feel this happening if you put your hand over your abdomen. In a few minutes, there is another contraction. With each one, the opening in the cervix is being made to spread or dilate, to allow the contents of the uterus to pass through to the vagina and out of you.

At first these contractions may be ten or fifteen minutes apart; but as they continue, they get closer together and each one lasts longer. Some women find them more uncomfortable than others. If they bother you a great deal, you can probably have a drug such as Demerol to relieve the pain. It may also help you to do the breathing exercise described in Chapter III—breathe deeply and regularly, in through your nose and out through your mouth. This helps you to relax, and it is something constructive you can do. It also speeds oxygen to the cramped muscles.

Several hours may go by before the cervix is fully dilated. Sometime during this period, the membranes of the amniotic sac may break, and you will feel a sploosh of warm liquid flowing out of your vagina. This seems to trigger some hormone related to labor; for after the sac breaks, the contractions come harder and closer together, which is good—the faster they come, the sooner it will be over.

When the cervix is dilated far enough, the uterus gives a few mighty heaves and pushes out its contents. You can definitely push, too, at this point. It's a little hard to describe, but when the time comes, you'll know how. Throughout your labor, you have been in your hospital bed, and you will expel the fetus into a bedpan. The placenta may come with it, or it may be expelled separately.

Afterward, you will be cleaned up and your bed changed, and a doctor will check to be sure that everything is out of your uterus. If the placenta has not been pushed out with the fetus, it may appear spontaneously within an hour or so. If it does not, you may be given a labor-inducing hormone to complete the abortion, or the material may be removed manually or with instruments.

Occasionally contractions do not begin even when 48 to 72 hours have elapsed since the saline injection. In that case, a second saline injection or some oxytocin may be used to bring on contractions.

Complications

The chief risks are that the saline solution may be injected somewhere other than in the amniotic sac; or that fetal material may be retained in the uterus, causing infection; or that a hemorrhage may occur after the placenta is expelled, at the place where it was attached to the uterus. Since the patient is in the hospital at the time symptoms of any of these problems appear, they can almost always be dealt with. Coping with them may be a quick and routine matter, or it may be frightening or painful; but none of these difficulties is likely to endanger your life. Also, the chance that any of them will actually occur at all is decreasing as doctors gain skill and experience in doing saline procedures.

One more risk has to be considered, though, when a saline abortion is done after the twentieth week. It is the tiny but devastating possibility that the fetus will be delivered alive. Because this chance exists, many hospitals are reluctant to perform abortions after this time. But the procedure is still entirely legal, and there is some evidence that saline abortions performed after twenty weeks may be slightly safer than those done earlier.

After a Saline Procedure

Once it is all over, you will probably stay in the hospital, and in bed, twelve to twenty-four hours for observation. If everything has gone well, you can then go home and resume normal activity.

Your postoperative instructions will be much the same as after an early abortion: take it easy for a day or two; don't do anything that could introduce germs into the vagina for at least two weeks; report fever of over 100° or any excessive cramps, pain, or bleeding at once; and have a checkup in two weeks. Your normal period should return in four to eight weeks.

If you have been properly supported and counseled throughout the experience, you should expect to feel great relief, and no more depression than you can cope with. It would be unrealistic to expect no down feeling at all. Knowing that some depression is natural may help you to deal with it. But heroics are not called for —and in this situation they may not be good for you. If you feel your emotions getting out of hand, talk to a friend or relative who understands your situation. Or call Planned Parenthood or the Clergy Consultation Service or your local Health Department; they will put you in touch with a counselor or social worker with whom you can discuss your feelings.

Hysterotomy

A hysterotomy is another kind of late abortion technique, but one rarely used. It is considered major surgery, and is usually performed only if other methods of abortion are ruled out for medical reasons, or if the patient wants to have a sterilization procedure done at the same time as the abortion. It must be done in a hospital under general anesthesia and requires several days' convalescence, so the bill is likely to be considerable. Hysterotomies cost at least $800 and can go a lot higher.

In performing the operation, the doctor makes a slit or incision low on the patient's abdomen, and the fetus and placenta are removed through this opening. When the incision heals, it tends to leave a weakened place in the wall of the uterus. Since this might well cause the uterus to split open during labor contractions, any children the woman has later will probably have to be delivered by Caesarean section. Remember that hysterotomy is not the same as hysterectomy, or removal of the uterus—it does *not* end fertility, unless a sterilization procedure is deliberately combined with it.

5

Controlling Your Fertility

In the aftermath of an abortion most women experience a variety of emotions. Most feel vastly relieved and consider themselves lucky to have been able to get a safe, legal abortion. Many also feel tense or sad or angry about the inconvenience, expense, and emotional strain involved. Almost all of them don't want to go through it again.

When you are first facing the crisis of unplanned pregnancy and the thought of abortion, you have to think through some subtle and complicated aspects of yourself as a woman and a sexual person in order to come to a decision you feel is right for you. After an abortion, when you come to contemplate the best way to avoid getting into that situation again, you have to think through a lot of the same questions. But now your situation is somewhat different. For one thing, if you never knew it before, you now know for sure that you are a fertile woman; and you realize with stunning clarity what the consequences of your fertility can be.

Some women are able to say to themselves, "OK, I know I am fertile, and that is good to know even if I learned it painfully. I now have a good reason to try to prevent conception when I don't want to be pregnant. But if the method I choose happens to fail, I know that abortion is available to me, and I know I can cope."

Others find that having an abortion has, to some extent, changed them as women and sexual people. What they feel they have learned through having one abortion is that they want never to have another—that they can't go through it again or, more subtly, that they can't be comfortable if they think of themselves as women who run around having abortions at the drop of a hat.

If you feel this way, yet you want to continue a normal and enjoyable sex life, your feeling may have a number of ramifications. First, it is a pretty strong incentive for choosing one of the contraceptive methods that have the highest rate of success. But it may be hard for you to feel 100 percent confidence in a method that has less than a 100 percent success rate, and none of them carries a guarantee. This can lead to a nagging fear in the back of your mind that it is going to fail and you will be trapped this time if it does—which in turn can erode or even destroy your ability to have and enjoy sex. In such a case, your best choice may simply be the method you *feel* most positive about (and to hell with the statistics), or you might even want to use two methods at once.

Some women decide to control future fertility by simply resolving never to have sex again. This is a perfectly valid option open to them; after all, a lot of single women are pressured into having sex they don't want. Some men use the very existence of contraceptives to pressure women to have sex—they argue that if you aren't afraid of getting pregnant, you have no excuse for refusing. That sword cuts two ways, both of them wrong. First, using contraceptives doesn't mean you aren't afraid of getting pregnant. Second, you don't *need* an excuse for refusing—if you don't want to, that's enough.

On the other hand, deciding not to choose a contraceptive method because you are determined never to have sex again is generally more complicated than that, and it is a decision which above all others must be examined very closely. There is a world of difference between not wanting sex and feeling you *shouldn't* want it.

Sometimes the rejection of contraception comes from a woman's feeling that if she keeps a contraceptive method available "in case," she will be more likely sooner or later to do what she thinks she ought not to. Or she may feel that just the planning ahead makes her guilty whether she has sex again or not. Or perhaps she feels that if she has sex she doesn't deserve protection —that she *should* have to suffer for it.

If such conflicting and guilty emotions are pulling at you, it may help to talk to a trained, objective counselor about them. Some women find it useful just to learn that there are people who don't feel her sexual nature is wicked. Others may at least come to recognize that if they have feelings of doubt and guilt, they can live with them without inflicting upon themselves the additional fear and danger of repeated unwanted pregnancy.

Contraception: Temporary Methods

No method is perfect for everybody; no single one is "best." You can only try to choose the one you feel is best for you—that will give you the highest level of protection with the least interference with your health *or* your sexual activity. This means, among other things, thinking realistically about your feelings about sex, and about the nature of your sex life—the conditions under which you make love, with whom, and how often.

The methods available are grouped here in order of effectiveness—the most successful first. But even the ones with higher failure rates work for some people; and if you strongly prefer one of them, it may work for you a lot better than a near-perfect method you hate. You have to use a method consistently and correctly for it to work, and realistically, you have to like it to use it.

Abstinence

As you know, conception can only occur when an egg in the woman's body is met and fertilized by a sperm from the man's. Avoiding sexual intercourse is therefore a prime way of preventing a meeting of sperm and egg. It is also the only one that can be guaranteed 100 percent effective. But this method only works if you *never* have sex—and never means *never*.

The Pill

After abstinence, the next most effective method is the Pill or, more accurately, the Pills.

Normally, as you are aware, a fertile woman's body releases an egg every month. But there are also times when this process is turned off naturally—when she is pregnant and during the first weeks when she is breast-feeding. At such times, her body's hormone level stays steadily high; as a result, her pituitary gland never gets the signal that would tell it to start the new cycle of hormone production that would result in ovulation—the release of an egg.

The Pill works on the same principle. It uses synthetic hormones like the ones produced by your body to fake the hormone levels of pregnancy and thus prevent ovulation. The Pill also affects the lining of the uterus so that even if an egg were to be released and fertilized it could not easily implant itself in the uterus, and it slightly alters the secretions in the cervix, making it less easy for sperm to penetrate.

The two basic kinds of Pill are called Combination and Sequential. The Combination type has two hormones, estrogen and pregesterone, in each pill. The Sequential has only estrogen in the first fifteen or sixteen pills and both estrogen and progesterone in the last five. The Sequential is less often prescribed than the Combination, because it seems to have a slightly higher rate of failure. It also provides a higher dose of estrogen than some Combination Pills, and estrogen is what is responsible for most of the undesirable side effects women may experience from the Pill.

You begin taking the Pill on Day 5 of a normal menstrual cycle, counting the first day of bleeding as Day 1. You then take one pill every day for twenty or

twenty-one days, as directed. (Most Pills now prescribed have twenty-one in the series.) Two days or so
after taking the last pill in the month's package, you
begin to menstruate and a new cycle begins; on Day 5
you begin taking the Pill again. Thus, if you take your
last Pill on a Friday, you theoretically begin to bleed on
Sunday, and take your next Pill on the following Friday. That way you always begin and end on the same
day of the week. For women who find it confusing to
stop and start at the right time, there are Pills packaged
with seven placebos, or fake Pills, for you to take during
the week of your period; that way you just have to
remember to swallow a Pill a day every day with no
break in routine.

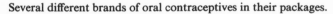

Several different brands of oral contraceptives in their packages.

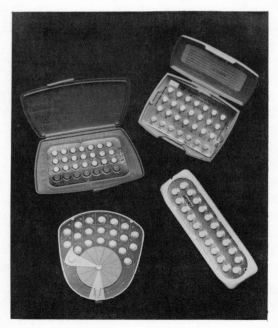

For the Pill to work, you have to remember to take it. No one pill protects you; it is the day-by-day action of the whole series that prevents ovulation all month long. Most people find it helps to get into a routine and stick to it, taking the Pill at the same time each day until it becomes a habit. They generally come in packages specially labeled to help you remember. If you usually take your Pill at bedtime, then when you get up in the morning you can check to make sure you didn't forget. If on Thursday morning you find Wednesday's pill still in the package, you take it then; that night you take your Thursday pill and you are still protected for the month. If on Thursday morning you find both the Tuesday and Wednesday pills still in the package, you take them as soon as you realize you have forgotten. Then you go on taking the rest of the pills, one each night, to prevent your cycle's getting mucked up; but you are no longer protected for sure, so you should also use an additional method of contraception for the rest of the month.

The advantage of the Pill is that it works. Provided they take it regularly only a very small fraction of one percent of women on the Pill get pregnant. Another great advantage is that it allows spontaneity in sex; you don't have to interrupt lovemaking to use it, and it allows you to feel more confident about sex because you are virtually sure you won't get pregnant.

But the Pill also has disadvantages. Some women find it simply impossible to remember every day. Others experience undesirable side effects. Since the Pill simulates pregnancy, some women actually feel such early pregnancy symptoms as nausea and fatigue for a month or two. The nausea can often be corrected by taking the Pill at mealtime; in any case, these symptoms generally go away after your body adjusts to its new arrangement of hormones.

A few women have more serious side effects that don't go away. These include migraine headache, weight gain, or blood clots (thromboembolism). The last is fairly rare, but very dangerous, and sometimes fatal. Sometimes minor side effects can be corrected simply by switching to another brand of pill. In other cases, the woman will have to stop taking the Pill altogether and at once.

Since there *are* possible risks and sideeffects, never borrow pills from a friend. The Pill should *never* be taken without a thorough examination by a doctor and the taking of a complete medical history, such as you had on the day of your abortion. The Pill will almost certainly be ruled out if you have ever had blood clots or inflammation of the veins, serious liver disease, or cancer of the breast or uterus. It may or may not be ruled out, depending on your own individual case, if you have heart disease, kidney disease, high blood pressure, diabetes, epilepsy, fibroids of the uterus, migraine headaches, serious visual problems, or severe depressions.

Some doctors don't tell their patients much about the risks and side effects of the Pill. First, because the danger *is* small, and because it is so much less than the physical (not to mention emotional) danger of pregnancy, which it prevents more successfully than any other method, they feel the risk is worth it—but then they aren't the ones taking the risks. Another reason doctors don't always tell you about side effects of the Pill is that they feel if they tell you you might have headaches, you *will* have headaches. And that is a valid point; plenty of people are very suggestible on the subject of aches and pains, especially if they've been told a lot of spooky stories.

Anyway, bear in mind that the vast majority of women get along fine with the Pill, so you shouldn't be looking for trouble. And if you experience headaches, weight gain and so on, you should be quite sure your symptoms aren't caused by the flu or overeating before you deprive yourself of an exceptionally reliable method of contraception. But if you do experience persistent or alarming side effects, by all means report them to a doctor; and if she or he doesn't take you seriously, find another doctor.

If you stop taking the Pill because of side effects, they will probably disappear almost at once. If you stop because you want to get pregnant, you will probably be ovulating normally within three months. There have been cases of couples who have not been able to have children after use of the Pill; but it is hard to say how many, if any, of these fertility problems were caused by the Pill, since 15 percent of couples are infertile temporarily or permanently anyway.

While on the Pill, you should have a semiannual or annual checkup that includes careful examination of the breast and Pap smears of the cervix. (Actually, you should have such a checkup every year even if you're not on the Pill.) Some doctors also suggest that patients go off the Pill periodically as a precaution against any unknown long-term effects of substituting synthetic hormone mechanisms for the body's own, over long periods of time.

The Mini-Pill

This is a new kind of oral contraceptive that has recently come on the market, finally approved by the Food and Drug Administration after several years of study.

The Mini-Pill contains synthetic progesterone only and works on a different principle from the Pill. In the majority of cases, it does not suppress ovulation; instead it acts primarily on the cervical secretions, making them hostile to sperm.

The Mini-Pill is taken every day of the year, which may be a convenience if you think you may get mixed up on the three-weeks-on, one-week-off schedule of the Pill. On the other hand, if you forget one pill, there is a greater chance of pregnancy than with conventional oral contraceptives. Even if you don't forget any, the chance of pregnancy is significantly greater—the failure rate of the Mini-Pill has been running about 3 percent.

The chief advantage of the new pill is supposed to be the complete absence of estrogen. But a small fraction of its progesterone content is converted in the body to biologically active estrogens; so the question of whether Mini-Pills have mini-risks, compared with conventional pills, is still not entirely settled. A disadvantage is the fact that some women who use the Mini-Pill tend to have unpredictable bleeding patterns—irregular periods and between-period spotting—even after prolonged use.

IUD

The Intrauterine Device—a device placed inside your

uterus—is another highly effective method of contraception that does not interfere with the act of lovemaking. IUDs come in different shapes, and are usually made of plastic. Of the many kinds available, the Lippes Loop seems to have the highest success rate with a minimum of problems. There are also newer smaller ones being tested, which are especially good for women who haven't had children; some use metals such as copper, which seems to have an additional backup effect in preventing pregnancy.

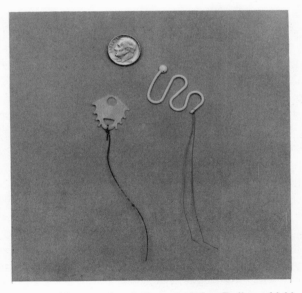

Two types of intrauterine devices: At left a Dalkon shield; at right, a Lippes loop. The dime gives an idea of their sizes.

No one knows exactly how, or why, the IUD works. The most popular current theories are that the IUD somehow causes the egg to travel through the Fallopian tube so fast that the fertilized egg is not yet ready to implant itself when it arrives in the uterus, or that the IUD affects the lining of the uterus in such a way as to prevent implantation. Anyway, they do seem to work for about 97 out of 100 women who can keep them in, which may make them about the greatest mystery medicine since aspirin (nobody knows how that works, either.)

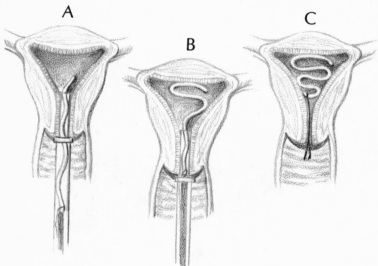

Three stages of insertion of a Lippes loop. At A the device is being inserted through a hollow plunger. At B the loop is beginning to uncoil in the uterus. At C the device is in place in the uterus with the threads extending just a slight distance beyond the cervix into the vagina.

An IUD is inserted in your uterus by a doctor. This can be done at any time. It is easiest when the cervical opening is slightly dilated—after an abortion or childbirth, or during your period. The device is straightened and compressed into a thin plastic tube that is inserted into the uterus. A plunger pushes the device out of the tube and it springs back into its original shape inside your uterus, touching the walls at several points. There it stays until you have a doctor remove it, unless by chance your body rejects it. Most IUDs have a tiny nylon thread attached to them that sticks out of the cervix into the vagina just far enough to be felt. This is so that every week or so, and certainly after every period, you can test with a finger in the vagina to see if the thread is still there. Sometimes you can't feel it because your uterus has bobbled into a tilted position that day. If you still can't find the strings after a few days, check with a doctor; it may be necessary to have an X-ray to be sure the IUD is still where it should be.

One important advantage of an IUD is that it doesn't interfere with your body chemistry—there are no side effects, except for rare cases of pelvic infection. Also, it doesn't interfere with sex.

A disadvantage is that about 35 percent of the women who try an IUD can't keep it—either the body rejects it, or the woman has to have it taken out because it makes her uncomfortable. Almost everybody feels some cramping for a few hours after the IUD is put in; in some cases severe cramps and heavy bleeding during periods last for several months. Sometimes if you have trouble with one kind of IUD, you will be able to tolerate another perfectly well; so if you have complaints, consider making a trade. Some people have back pain or breakthrough bleeding between periods; and these symptoms, too, can often be corrected by switching to another shape of IUD.

In theory, the IUD is effortless as well as effective protection. But you do have to check regularly to make sure you haven't pushed it out. Some women also worry about that 3 percent failure rate, which is out of their control—the IUD is the only method of contraception that protects or fails without action on your part—but you can provide some extra insurance, if you want to, by using an additional contraceptive such as spermicidal foam.

The Diaphragm, with Spermicidal Cream or Jelly

The diaphragm is a cap made of thin rubber that fits over your cervix, blocking the opening between the vagina and the uterus. It is used with a special cream or jelly that kills sperm, so the method works two ways —it blocks the sperm physically *and* chemically. You put it in yourself before having sex, but you must be

Two sizes of diaphragm, with one type of the jelly or cream that should be used with this contraceptive device.

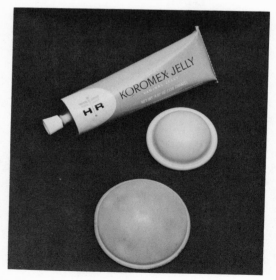

fitted for it by a doctor—women come in all different sizes. When you are fitted, the doctor explains how to use the diaphragm and shows you how to put it in; after that it's up to you.

Before making love—just before, or several hours ahead—you smear the diaphragm on both sides with the spermicidal cream or jelly. The rubber of the diaphragm is stretched over a flexible metal ring with a spring in it. To insert, you fold the ring in half and slide it well into your vagina with your fingers or a special inserter, and when you let go, it springs open, covering the opening of the uterus with a thin layer of rubber and spermicide. It is completely comfortable when it is in place and it stays by itself; it can't fall out, and you can't feel it. If you make love more than three hours after putting it in, add more cream or jelly to your vagina just before sex. If you make love more than once, add more cream before each of the man's orgasms.

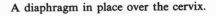

A diaphragm in place over the cervix.

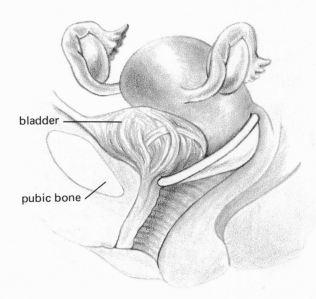

bladder

pubic bone

After sex, you wait at least six hours before taking the diaphragm out. This is to maintain the barrier to the uterus as long as some sperm might still be alive and lurking in the vagina. You then remove the diaphragm by dislodging the rim with a finger or the hook of an inserter and sliding it out. You wash it well, dry it, and put it away covered with talcum powder or cornstarch to keep the rubber from drying and cracking.

The advantages of the diaphragm are that it causes no pain or side effects of any kind, and it works splendidly *if* it is used right. A possible disadvantage is that it is not constantly with you like the Pill or IUD; you have to use it every time you have intercourse, and that means you must either stop in the middle of making love or else plan ahead enough to put it in beforehand. But sometimes there is no way of knowing that you are going to have sex; or you may be afraid it will look calculating for you to have put in a diaphragm or even brought one. So the diaphragm may not be an ideal method for those who do not have a comfortable relationship and understanding with their partner or partners, or those who have sex at unpredictable times and places. It may also turn off a woman who feels uncomfortable about touching her genitals.

Condoms

Also called a rubber, a prophylactic or a "safety," the condom is a very easy and very reliable method. It is a sheath of very thin rubber which fits over the erect penis like a stocking and prevents the sperm from swimming off into the vagina. It is put on during lovemaking, by you or the man, *before* the penis enters the vagina, not just before orgasm. Long before the man comes, he may release droplets of semen containing particularly energetic sperm, and if the penis is in the vagina or just outside it, pregnancy can well result. After ejaculation, the man withdraws his penis before it completely relaxes, holding the top of the condom in place so it won't slip or spill. A fresh condom is needed for each ejaculation.

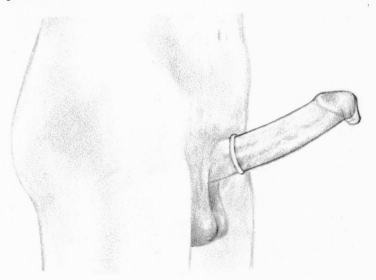

A condom worn correctly. Note that the tip of the condom forms a "reservoir."

Condoms are made of very thin rubber or animal membrane in order to interfere with sensation as little as possible. When putting the condom on, it is important to leave about half an inch of space at the tip so the semen will have somewhere to go. If it is put on too tightly or if air gets inside, the pressure of ejaculation could split the condom. Fancy ones have "reservoir tips"—little toes at the end for the semen; some also have special lubricants. All American-made brands offered in drug stores and family planning centers are quality-tested against standards set by the government, so you get the same protection no matter what you pay.

The advantages of the condom are that they are inexpensive and available in any drugstore; they carry no risks or side effects for either the man or the woman; they provide protection against both pregnancy and VD (the only method that does both); and they are small and convenient to carry with you. Just be sure to keep them in their protective foil wrappings so that the rubber doesn't dry and crack. Since condoms may become defective in their old age, you should also beware of those sold in vending machines. They have been subjected to the same tests as others, but you have no way of knowing how long they have been sitting in the machine; and if the machine is exposed to sun or heat or cold, they may deteriorate.

The condom's disadvantages are that many men feel it cuts down their enjoyment of sex and some men resent having any responsibility for contraception whatever. They can also feel dry and tight in the vagina. But if you want additional lubrication you can try using one of the vaginal spermicidal products; this will also provide the bonus of extra protection. Don't use Vaseline, though—it's no good for rubber.

Vaginal Foams, Creams, and Jellies

These products are spermicides—sperm killers—that are inserted in the vagina just before intercourse. They are a lot better than nothing, but not as effective as the Pill, the IUD, diaphragms, or condoms. You buy them at a drug store without a prescription. Foam comes in an aerosol can, and cream and jelly come in tubes; each has a plastic plunger which helps you measure the right amount and get it into the upper vagina at the cervix. In place, they form a foamy or creamy cap over the cervix which (ideally) blocks and kills the sperm before it can enter the uterus.

Used with an IUD, diaphragm, or condom, they make the combination nearly fail-safe; used alone, spermicides are less successful. In any case, they have to be used during or immediately before lovemaking (not more than an hour before, preferably thirty minutes) and a fresh application must be used before each ejaculation. They involve you in no risks (except the risk of pregnancy) and have no side effects except an occasional irritation to a penis or vagina. This clears up as soon as you wash or douche, but you shouldn't do either until eight hours after making love. If you or the man have an allergic reaction to one brand, you can usually clear it up by switching to another.

Vaginal Foaming Tablets

These, too, are sold in drug stores, without a prescription, and you put them into the vagina way up at the cervix. The tablet must be wet when you put it in place in order for it to foam up and form a chemical barrier to sperm. The barrier is supposed to be the equivalent of what you would get with aerosol foam; but the tablet is less easy to insert than foam, and timing is trickier— you have to wait no less than five minutes before making

love (to give the tablet time to fizz) but no more than
half an hour. Still, if you don't mind making love by the
clock, they are better than nothing.

Vaginal Suppositories

Also sold in drug stores without prescription, these
are little waxy lumps that contain a spermicide. If you
put one in the upper vagina at the cervix no less than
fifteen (and no more than thirty) minutes before intercourse, it will supply some protection against conception—that is, if it melts. But it won't provide much; and
if your timing is off, or the suppository doesn't melt for
reasons of its own, it won't give any protection at all
worth mentioning.

Withdrawal (Coitus Interruptus)

Withdrawal has been with us for a long time—long
enough to have a name from the classical Latin. It
means interrupting intercourse before ejaculation; the
man withdraws his penis from the vagina before he
comes. Its main advantage is that it is free and readily
available if you have run out of everything else and all
the drug stores are closed, and if you cannot possibly
wait till tomorrow night for genital intercourse.

But the risk of pregnancy is great, because of those
drops of semen that emerge from the penis well before
actual orgasm; and because of the self-control necessary
by the man. Even if no sperm are deposited inside the
vagina, they may make their way in from outside, if
ejaculation occurs close enough to the opening of the

vagina, and if the area is well enough lubricated to give the sperm something to swim in. Withdrawal also tends to interfere with the enjoyment of sex for both the man and the woman, especially if it is the only method used by a couple for a long period of time.

Rhythm

This method is based on the natural *rhythm* of the woman's menstrual cycle. It involves determining when in your cycle ovulation occurs, then abstaining from sex for about four days before (because sperm can live for days in the uterus, just waiting for an unsuspecting egg) and a couple of days after (because the egg can live in the Fallopian tube up to 36 hours). The difficulties of this method—and it *is* difficult—are knowing when you are "safe" in the first place, and then faithfully refraining from sex on the "unsafe" days.

Rhythm can work, but only if it is practiced faithfully and with a doctor's advice, and if the woman is fairly regular in her menstrual cycle. It is used by many Roman Catholic couples because it is the only method accepted by the Church. Many couples only *think* they are using it, however. Knowing vaguely that there are "unsafe" days in the middle of the cycle, they abstain for a couple of days two weeks after the period—but actually practicing Rhythm is a good deal more complicated than that.

In a textbook regular cycle, ovulation occurs about fourteen days *before* the next period. Knowing when that will be is like saying to a stranger on a bus, "Watch me and get off one stop before I do." To make anything like an accurate prediction you have to keep a careful written record of the starting dates of your periods for several months—the more the better.

In addition, a doctor will usually ask you to keep a record of your basal body temperature every day for several months. This requires a special thermometer; and the temperature taking must be done the first thing in the morning, before you get up, sit up, or speak. From these records, the doctor can then help you calculate your own particular set of "safe" and "unsafe" days.

As noted, this method cannot really be used without the help of a doctor or family planning clinic—to show you how to keep the necessary records and to interpret your particular pattern. Even then it is never more than highly educated guesswork; and even if you guess right, there is still the problem of two persons' will power functioning just right, all the time.

Nonmethods

Some of the foregoing methods, as you have gathered, work very well for almost everybody, and some work for fewer people; but if you have been using something not so far described it almost surely doesn't work at all.

Douching doesn't work, homemade condoms don't work, having sex in different positions doesn't work. Feminine hygiene products are for cleanliness, not contraception. A lot of women are particularly confused about these items because they see advertisements for hygiene sprays promising "feminine freshness," and advertisements for suppositories that offer to "control intimate problems." But if a package of suppositories isn't clearly labeled "for contraception," don't just buy something and hope—call a family planning clinic and find out.

One poignant misconception is that some people imagine a woman, like a man, must have an orgasm for pregnancy to occur. This is definitely not true—your pleasure has nothing to do with it, and you accomplish nothing but frustration by avoiding orgasm. More women than you probably want to hear about have had baby after baby, and never an orgasm in their lives.

Where to Get Contraceptive Devices and Information

If you have chosen a method requiring a prescription and you don't have a private doctor, call Planned Parenthood, or the family planning clinic at a local hospital for information and/or service.

Contraception: Permanent Methods

If you are quite sure you want no more children, or no children at all, you can have your fertility permanently ended by voluntary sterilization. You should understand that sterilization is not reversible. There *have* been cases in which the operations were successfully undone, but you can't count on it; and you should not opt for sterilization with any notion that you can later change your mind and become fertile again.

Vasectomy

For a man, sterilization is a relatively quick, simple procedure that can be done in a family planning clinic or in the office of a doctor, usually a urologist. It simply involves cutting each vas deferens— the two tubes that transport the sperm from the testicles into the semen. Afterwards, the man will have all the same sexual desires and responses he always did; he will have erections and ejaculations exactly as before. The only difference is that no sperm will be in the semen, and so no pregnancy can result.

The procedure usually involves at least three office visits to the clinic or doctor. In the first, the man discusses his decision with the doctor and has some tests, including a semen analysis. The second visit is for the operation, which begins with an injection into the scrotum of a local anesthetic like Novocaine. When the area is numb, a small incision is made in each scrotal sac. First on one side, then on the other, the doctor draws out the vas deferens, ties it in two places with a piece of thread, then cuts the tube between the tie-offs.

There have been a very few cases of these tubes growing back together by themselves—far too few for you to worry about. But you can imagine the havoc that follows when a man is sure he is sterile and his wife turns up pregnant; therefore you should at least know about the possibility—so that if the worst does happen, you will check with a doctor before you shoot each other.

After the vasectomy, the man returns to the doctor for sperm checks to be sure that there are no sperm in his semen. As a rule, several of these checks have to be made at monthly intervals before two successively sperm-free ones prove the operation has been a success.

He goes right on reproducing sperm in his testicles; they just don't get past the tie-off in the vas to reach the semen. Instead, they are absorbed by the body.

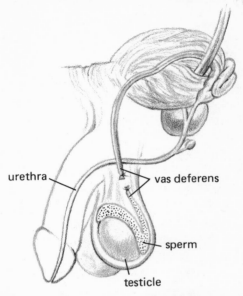

In a vasectomy, the vas deferens on each side is cut and tied, so that sperm cannot reach the fluid in the man's sexual discharge.

Vasectomy is highly effective, low-risk, minor surgery. It costs $150 or less at a clinic—somewhat more if it is done by a private doctor. Its possible disadvantages are the very small chance of a spontaneous reversal; and for some couples the fact that the woman is protected only if she has sex with that one man.

Occasionally, after a vasectomy, a man will worry so much about whether the operation can affect his sexual performance that the worry itself affects it. If a man has that kind of apprehension, he should certainly seek competent counseling before and, if necessary, after the operation. Perhaps he should not have the operation at all.

Tubal Ligation

For a woman, the most common form of sterilization is tubal ligation—the tying and cutting of her Fallopian tubes. This serves to prevent the egg from passing through the tube to the uterus each month, and prevents any sperm from passing up the tube past the point of ligation.

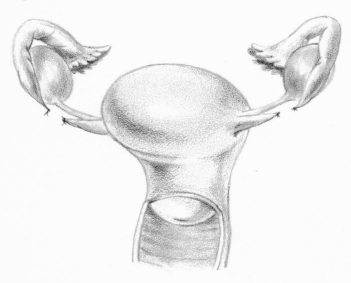

In a tubal ligation, the Fallopian tubes are tied and cut, preventing the passage of eggs into the uterus.

Done in the traditional way, it is considered major surgery, requiring general anesthesia and hospitalization. The doctor reaches the tubes through an incision in the abdomen; afterward several days of in-hospital recuperation are required; thus the whole thing is pretty expensive—at least $300, sometimes much more. It can be done at any time, but to minimize expense it is often done when a woman who wants it is still in the hospital after giving birth, or after a hysterotomy. Afterwards the woman will continue to ovulate and to have all her normal hormone functions and normal desires; the only difference is that the egg can't reach the sperm, and vice versa. Instead the released egg disintegrates each month and is absorbed by the body.

A new and much simpler technique of female sterilization using laparoscopy is being developed and used in some places. The doctor inserts a laparoscope—a narrow tube containing lights and mirrors—into the abdomen through a very small incision near the bellybutton. This enables him or her to see the Fallopian tubes without making a large cut. Through the same incision or another tiny one, slender instruments are inserted with which the tubes are held, cauterized (burned), closed, then cut. The great advantage of this technique is that it is not major surgery—it requires only a short hospital stay and may even be done on an out-patient basis. As a result, it takes less time to recover from, and costs much less than the older (and still more common) method of tubal ligation.

Getting a Sterilization Procedure

Until recently, some hospitals maintained a mystical

code to determine who is eligible for voluntary sterilization—your age multiplied by the number of your children had to work out to a certain number, so that if you
were forty and had no children or nineteen and had
three, you might not be able to make the decision for
yourself. Today, more and more hospitals have aban-
doned arbitrary formulas and evaluate each application
individually. But if you think or know you want sterilization and nevertheless run into hassles of the old kind,
you can call Planned Parenthood, or write the Associa-
tion for Voluntary Sterilization, 14 West 40th Street,
New York, N.Y. 10018, for the name of a doctor or
hospital who will serve you.

6

The Future of Fertility Control

The Medical Future

The medical future of abortion is a subject closely involved with the whole field of development and research in methods of birth control. Abortion is a form of birth control—probably the most widely used method on earth. But from a medical point of view, abortion is a less desirable procedure than avoiding conception in the first place, and from the woman's point of view this is truer still. So research goes on constantly to discover a more effective method of contraception than we have now—searching for pills for women and IUDs that will work without causing side effects, better spermicides, and so on. Some research (though not enough) is being done on contraceptive devices to be used by men.

But even if contraceptive methods are improved, even if information and devices are made more available and less expensive, there will always be a need for abortion as a method of birth control. There will always be contraceptives that fail, there will always be wanted pregnancies that turn out to endanger the woman's life, there will always be pregnancies that are planned and have to be unplanned because of a change in the woman's health or life situation, damage to the fetus, or some other reason. So research goes on to improve our present methods of abortion—to make it safer, less expensive, and less traumatic.

Recently a third area of research has opened up that bridges the gap between contraception and abortion— methods that chemically or mechanically work on the reproductive cycle during that gray period after conception has or has not occurred, but before pregnancy can be diagnosed. One you may have heard of is the "morning after" pill. This is a high dose of estrogen given for several days after unprotected intercourse. It is given orally or by injection not more than three days after intercourse, while the egg would still be traveling down the Fallopian tube. It affects the uterine lining so that *if* an egg has been released and fertilized, it will not be able to implant itself in the uterus when it arrives there, and conception will not be completed. Its drawback is that that much estrogen can give you the world's most horrendous case of morning sickness all day long, and that estrogen can also have other undesirable side effects, as described for the Pill in Ch. V. At present it is usually only given in an emergency such as rape; in any case it is hardly a method to choose for regular use.

Other experimental methods of contraception using hormones found in the Pill are a once-a-month Pill and a progesterone injection given every three months in a special long-lasting form. It is not clear yet how well these work, and they have side effects such as spotty bleeding between periods or no real period at the right time. Also, if you have a three-month injection and it makes you feel lousy, you're stuck with it for three months. But these are promising methods for those who can't remember a pill every day or who react badly to estrogen.

Another very promising discovery is prostaglandin— a hormone-like substance that can induce contractions of the uterus. It is named after the prostate gland, where semen is produced, because prostaglandins are present in male semen, as well as in many other parts of the body. It is also present in the uterus during menstruation, when the uterus contracts to let the blood flow out through the cervix, and in the amniotic fluid when the uterus contracts in abortion or full-term delivery—but not at other times. Experiments have determined that prostaglandins can *produce* contractions of the uterus —which means they could be used to bring on menstruation whether conception has occurred or not, or to push out the contents of the uterus at any stage of pregnancy. This would be especially valuable to the women seven weeks pregnant or less, for whom there is not currently an approved method of abortion, for the 13–15 weeks interim period when it is too late for curettage and too early for saline induction, and for any time thereafter. In a nonpregnant or early pregnant woman it can be placed in the vagina in tablet form; later, it can be injected into the amniotic fluid (as in a saline abortion). Prostaglandins work faster than saline solution—usually in 8–11 hours, but they can cause nausea, vomiting, or diarrhea, and certainly cramps. Research continues in order to learn how to control these side effects and how to administer the hormones best—in a vein, in the vagina, in the uterus, or in the amniotic sac. When the long-range effects of this method are known, and when and if the side effects can be controlled, prostaglandins could become a form of birth control to be administered by the woman routinely any month her period is late.

Something usually called "menses extraction" or "endometrial aspiration" is a technique that has been used for several years. Using a hand syringe and a thin flexible plastic tube, one can suck out the menses, or monthly shedding of the uterine lining. Since the tube is thin it can usually be used without dilating the cervix, and since it is flexible it offers less danger of perforation of the uterus than standard early abortion techniques. Menses extraction is done up to ten days after a period is missed—generally before any pregnancy test can show whether conception has occurred. But if a fertilized egg is present in the uterus, it will usually be sucked out along with the rest of the monthly shedding.

This technique is fast and relatively painless and can be done in a doctor's office, which makes it less traumatic and far less expensive than a standard early abortion; there is reason to believe that some doctors have been offering menses extraction as a form of illegal abortion for years. However it is not an established method of birth control because as yet there is no body of medical literature assessing its effectiveness, safety, and long-range effects.

The Legal Future of Abortion

Abortion has for some years been legal in many parts of the world, including England, Sweden, Japan, Bulgaria, Czechoslovakia, Hungary, and mainland China. On January 22, 1973, with a landmark Supreme Court decision in the cases of Roe v. Wade and Doe v. Bolton, the United States joined these countries. The court ruled 7–2 that in the first trimester no state may interfere in any way with a woman's decision to have an abortion as long as the abortion is performed by a physician. In the second trimester of pregnancy, the state may lay down medical guidelines as to where abortions may be performed, what emergency facilities must be available and so on, but only to protect the health of the woman. The state may not interfere with the actual decision to have the abortion. Only in the last trimester may a state ban abortions, and even then abortions may still be performed when there is danger to the life or health of the mother.

The majority opinion written by Justice Blackmun indicated that a woman's right to decide for herself whether to bear a child is guaranteed under the Fourteenth Amendment to the Constitution, the amendment which has been interpreted as a citizen's right to privacy. It explained that whatever the medical and theological opinions on the subject, an unborn human is not a person as defined by the Constitution, and that a fetus does not have Constitutional rights.

To conform to the Court's ruling, the laws of every state in the union except New York will have to be revised or entirely rewritten, and in the meantime the terms of the decision will effectively be the law of the land. This decision will mean a new era in the right of women to safe, dignified, legal abortion, but it would be naive to expect that the controversy is at an end. To understand the factors leading to the Court's action and to put in perspective the discussion as well as dissension that is still to come, it is important to review the opinions and events that have figured in the abortion controversy up to the present time.

At the time of the Court's ruling, fourteen states and the District of Columbia had reformed their anti-abortion laws to permit abortion under certain circumstances, such as danger to the woman's health, risk of fetal deformity, and cases of rape or incest. In some of these states, the law was liberally interpreted in such a way as to make abortion available virtually "on request"—if the woman wanted an abortion, it was considered that denying it constituted a threat to her mental health. In others, the law was interpreted very conservatively; a woman may have had to submit her case to a number of doctors and to a hospital review board, sometimes requiring the consent of as many as fourteen people besides herself and her doctor. The law was interpreted according to local politics and prejudices, and it was sometimes harder to get a legal abortion in a "reformed" state than an unreformed one. Unreformed states generally permitted abortion only when the mother's life was at stake. This could mean that if she threatened to kill herself her life was thought to be endangered; or it could mean that if pregnancy would leave her paralyzed or debilitated but not kill her, an abortion would be denied.

❲ In the meantime, three states—Alaska, Hawaii, and Washington—had liberalized their abortion laws to permit abortion on request, but only to women already living in the state and only up to a certain point, ranging from sixteen to twenty weeks. The abortion law in New York State conforms most closely to the ruling of the Supreme Court, so the experience of New York State in the past two years is especially relevant to any consideration of what we may expect throughout the nation.]

Since July 1, 1970, when New York's liberal abortion law went into effect, maternal death rates in New York State have plummeted. This is because many fewer women are dying of botched abortions performed by incompetent abortionists or by themselves, and also because many fewer women to whom full-term pregnancy is dangerous are being forced to continue their pregnancies. So death rates are lower for both septic abortions and for full-term deliveries.

Infant death rates are also at the lowest point they have ever been—again, because fewer women who are too young or too old or who have other health problems known to involve risks to the infants they carry, are being forced to continue pregnancies.

From 1954, when such records began to be kept, out-of-wedlock birthrates climbed higher and higher every year. But in 1970, the rate reversed. Statewide the rate has dropped 14.2 percent in two years.

Yet in the spring of 1972, the New York State legislature voted to repeal the new law and reinstate the old restrictive one, and only Governor Nelson Rockefeller's veto prevented their vote from becoming law. In spite of the obvious benefits of the law in terms of public health, and in spite of praise from public health officials and the President's Commission on Population Growth and the American Future, which termed the New York law a model and recommended that all other states liberalize their laws "along the lines of the New York State statute," they wanted to take it all back.

To help understand why, it is important to consider abortion in a context of historical, medical, and legal factors. In most cultures throughout most of history, a woman's right to have an abortion before the fetus quickened (about twenty weeks) was unquestioned. Quickening was thought of as the beginning of life, although we now know that it is simply the first point at which the woman can feel the fetus moving, not the moment it becomes alive and not even the first moment it moves. In 1829, when New York first passed a law forbidding abortion, except when the woman's life was in danger, it was not because abortion was thought morally wrong, but because it was terribly dangerous. Surgery of any kind was dangerous and the only reason all surgery was not outlawed was that no one would submit to any surgery unless he or she would definitely die without it. Later in the century other states passed laws outlawing abortion; surgery was becoming safer, but times were changing. The later laws had less to do with saving women's lives and more to do with prevailing attitudes about women and sex. The Victorian era had begun. Sex became a completely taboo subject, not to be talked of, hardly to be thought of. In such a climate, small wonder that abortion was outlawed.

Also, during the years when most of this country's anti-abortion legislation was enacted, America had a population problem. It needed more people. This fact, combined with prevailing attitudes toward sex, made prohibiting abortion seem the only thing to do—on the surface. In real life, of course, behind closed doors where society didn't have to see or think of it, abortions were going on as always (just as pregnancies were). The only difference was that abortions were no longer performed by doctors, but by criminal abortionists.

Women who could not afford an illegal abortionist or couldn't find one, turned to the most dangerous abortionists of all—themselves. They tried to end their pregnancies by drinking dangerous substances thought to be abortifacients, douching with lye solutions, or sticking sharp objects into their uteri, usually causing infection, perforation, sterility, or death.

Meanwhile, in places where abortions could be performed legally, medical advances had long since reversed the relative dangers of abortion and childbirth. (New York City's 1972 figures reflect this dramatically —29 maternal deaths for every 100,000 childbirths, as opposed to only 3.5 per 100,000 legal abortions.) So by the 1970's, laws that were originally intended to save women's lives were seen to be endangering them instead. Similarly, the population issue has reversed. America, and the world in general, needs to reduce its rate of population growth. Given these considerations, in the twentieth century it became increasingly possible to locate a doctor willing to perform an illegal abortion —*if* you had money, and *if* you knew somebody who knew somebody. More and more, anti-abortion laws were not preventing abortions—they were simply making them expensive and hard to find, and preventing the medical establishment from regulating and monitoring them. These are the conditions which led four states to repeal their anti-abortion laws, and twelve others to dramatically reform them by 1970.

From the point of view of the anti-abortionists, abortion is murder, because they believe that a human life is created at the moment of conception. Anyone who believes abortion is tantamount to taking an actual human life, will most probably reject abortion as a possibility for herself. However, it *is* a matter of personal opinion. Biologically, there is no one point at which life begins. Every egg a woman will release throughout her life is present and "alive" in her body when she is born, and every egg and sperm represents a potential person. The ancients felt that life became an actual person at the moment of quickening. Some, as noted, feel that it occurs at conception, and others feel that personhood accrues gradually day by day over forty weeks of gestation. Since it is in fact a question of life, it is small wonder that opinions are strongly held and deeply felt. What has been surprising is the fact that a minority tried to make its personal opinion legal and binding for all of us—thereby denying the rest of the population the right to reach its own decision.

But we wonder if the issue of abortion as murder is the only issue. After all, no one suggested actually making it punishable as murder—they were content with making it dangerous, expensive, and discriminatory. Wasn't the issue—isn't it still—the right and ability of women seeking abortions to decide for themselves? Wasn't the legislature really saying that they mistrusted the *reasons* women are seeking abortions? Perhaps it was the very success of liberalized abortion that caused second thoughts. Because if it *is* safe, if it is available on the same basis as all other medical services—then what? What does that mean for our sexual mores? For the moral fabric of society? For law and order? If illicit sex doesn't have dangerous consequences, what is to keep everyone from doing it?

Abortion is unlike other medical issues *because* it is connected in our minds with sex—and especially with illicit sex. It is no use declaiming that almost as many married women as single seek abortions; none of us is entirely rational about sex, or abortion; not the legislators, not the pro or anti pressure groups, not women seeking abortions. A life-and-death issue combined with a sex-in-the-streets issue is bound to be emotional and political dynamite. We all need to examine ourselves and our motives very carefully to learn *why* we stand *where* we stand; facing our most deeply held beliefs about sex and abortion is at least as subtle and complex as interpreting Constitutional guarantees—and that's going some.

Somewhere deep in ourselves we all think that unbridled sexuality is wrong for somebody. We may think it is bad for teen-agers, we may think it is bad for the unmarried, we may think it is bad, period. Somewhere all of us draw the line. Now if we think it is bad, and if we think it is going on, then somewhere in our hearts we think something should be done about it, but we aren't sure what. Maybe more sex education would help, maybe no sex education would help—and maybe fear of illegal abortion would help.

It is easy to see why someone who has never had an abortion may think that the idea that abortion is "easy" makes irresponsible sex more inviting, but there are flaws in that train of thought. First, there is absolutely no indication that abortion, even at its most terrifying, ever acted as a deterrent to sex. If the very real danger and difficulty of illegal abortion didn't deter women from seeking such abortions—and it didn't—then how could it be said to deter them from having sex? But the second flaw, the more important one, is the notion that abortion is easy. Health workers, social workers, counselors, and doctors, after two years of legal abortion in New York, have suggested that there is almost no such thing as a woman who decides to have an abortion without soul-searching. The fact that there are fewer devastating psychological aftereffects to legal abortion than illegal abortion, as noted in Chapter 3, to some of us indicates one thing; that women are devoting their emotional energy to examining the real moral and social implications of their pregnancy and their abortion, rather than to stealth, conniving, and law-breaking as they were forced to when abortion was illegal. That, some feel, was a real threat to the emotional and moral health of the woman and of society.

But, others wonder, how can we know that the availability of abortion isn't breeding a new kind of contempt for sexual mores? How can we know that the women who have sought abortions have done so responsibly and with due consideration? There is no answer. If you have had an abortion, you know what it meant to you. If you have decided against it, that in itself indicates that the availability of abortion did not make it an "easy out" for you. Perhaps a more relevant consideration is, if abortions are *illegal,* who are the women who manage to get them safely anyway? Are they young, inexperienced, ignorant? The woman in menopause who didn't know she was still fertile? The married woman who can't afford a fifth child? Not likely. Illegal abortions are available to the women who can afford them and to those who know where to get them. That is, to women who can buy their way out of a predicament, and to women who are familiar with that particular path of law-breaking, who know people who have done it before, or who have done it before themselves. That doesn't mean it was easy for them; there was still guilt and fear, there were no guarantees that if something went wrong they wouldn't be sent home to fester or hemorrhage, or left in the street. Even if nothing went wrong, there was the pain, since illegal abortions are often performed without anesthetic. Abortion is never easy. But if the question is the moral health of society, it is hard to see how the experience of illegal abortion contributes to it.

As abortion laws now stand, no woman need have one; no doctor need perform one. Those who do want abortions are free to decide this most crucial, intimate, and private issue according to their own personal deeply held beliefs. There are those who fear that allowing the termination of any potential life will lead to a diminished respect for the value of all life. This is certainly a serious question, one we cannot afford to ignore. In the countries where abortion has been legal for some time there is no indication that such a thing has come to pass. But in considering this elusive question, this matter of the damage to the spirit caused by allowing or forbidding abortion, we must remember to consider the psychological damage done to a woman who is forced to have an illegal abortion, or to have an unwanted child. What can be her feelings toward a society that denies her the right to make such a decision for herself? .What does that say to her about the value society places on her and her life?

Certainly, abortion puts an end to one potential human life. But unwanted births can pose just as real a threat to life. They can damage irretrievably the future of the mother; damage her ability to nurture the children she has, perhaps end forever the possibility of her having loved and wanted children at some other, better time in her life. There is also high risk to the quality of life of the unwanted child. When a woman bears a child under coercion, against her own best judgment and perhaps the judgment of her doctor, when she is not prepared or equipped to care for one, too often the child is seen as a punishment, and is punished in turn. The child may suffer crippling material and emotional deprivation; every year, children born to parents who cannot cope with them are, quite literally, physically battered as well.

Perhaps the most important thing to realize is that at this point in time, abortion is not only a moral issue; it is a political issue. Morally, we each decide for ourselves whether abortion is right or wrong; whether it is a simplistic case of taking a life or whether it is a more complex matter of weighing the rights of a potential person against the rights of an actual one. But we must also face the political issue—the question of whether we are also prepared to let others decide. If after reading this book you conclude that abortion is not the right alternative for you, you realize what a deeply personal, individual matter that decision is. If you have decided to have an abortion you have probably come through the experience with a better understanding of yourself as a woman, and of the importance of accepting responsibility for your fertility. Certainly you have been exposed to a great deal of information about fertility and birth control which will help you to make your own decisions most effectively in the future. But you may believe that abortion is fundamentally wrong, not only for you, but for everyone. If so, your right to advocate that attitude, to persuade others to believe as you do, is protected under present abortion laws.

The matter of if and when to bear a child is delicate, complex, and profoundly important to the woman involved, and to us all—so important that it ought to be considered carefully and specifically each time an unwanted pregnancy occurs, not controlled by an arbitrary and unspecific policy laid down by the state.

With the legal battle over the right to abortion apparently at an end, women are at last free to reach their own decisions on this matter in an informed, responsible way, with dignity, and with a belief in their right and ability to do so. But while we are at the beginning of a new era, we have by no means seen the last of the old one. There will surely continue to be conflict, confusion, and resentment toward the notion of abortions among those who oppose them, and even among those who will have them.

But for many others, abortion can now become what it should be—at the least, a safe medical procedure; at the best, a constructive, instructive, growing experience. Never again in America need abortion be a source of fear or shame. It has become a matter of free choice about the quality of life—our own lives and the lives of our children.

Where to Call

When this book went to press (April, 1973), the listings that follow were accurate, but don't be surprised if you find that some numbers have changed. If you run into a problem, check with "Information" in the city listed, or call the national headquarters of either Planned Parenthood or the Clergy Consultation Service. Both are in New York City. The Clergy number is (212) 477-0034; Planned Parenthood's is (212) 541-7800.

If you live in Arkansas, Louisiana, North or South Dakota, or Wyoming, you won't find any numbers listed for your state. See what the listings have to offer in neighboring states and call the agency nearest you; or phone the numbers given in the first paragraph. Other local sources of help may be the Department of Health in your city, county, or state; or your college health service, if you're a student.

If you are not a resident of New York City but have decided, for whatever reason, that you'd prefer to go there for an abortion, the number to call is (212) 677-3040—the Family Planning Information Service. This is the city's central source for abortion referrals—to clinics, hospitals, or private physicians. FPIS makes no charge for information or referrals and will not refer you to any facility whose services have been found to be unsatisfactory.

CLERGY CONSULTATION SERVICES

ALABAMA	Birmingham	(205) 887-7182
	Mobile	(205) 479-4429
ARIZONA		(602) 967-4234
COLORADO		(303) 757-4442
CONNECTICUT		(203) 624-8646
FLORIDA	Gainesville	(305) 372-5883
	Jacksonville	(904) 354-2817
	Tampa	(813) 933-5031
ILLINOIS	Champaign	(217) 352-1203
	Chicago	(312) 667-6015
	Peoria	(309) 676-4126
INDIANA		(219) 422-2288
IOWA		(515) 282-1738

KANSAS		(913) 539-3011
LOUISIANA		(504) 897-6980
MAINE		(207) 773-3866
MASSACHUSETTS		(413) 586-3478
MICHIGAN	Detroit	(313) 964-0838
	Grand Rapids	(616) 454-2693
	Lansing	(517) 332-6410
MINNESOTA		(612) 545-8085
MISSISSIPPI		(601) 362-7075
NEBRASKA		(402) 453-5314
NEW HAMPSHIRE		(603) 646-2558
NEW JERSEY		(201) 933-2937
NEW YORK		(212) 477-0034
NORTH CAROLINA		(919) 967-5333
OHIO	Cincinnati	(513) 721-1015
	Cleveland	(216) 229-7423
	Columbus	(614) 224-5008
	Dayton	(513) 278-6144
	Toledo	(419) 243-9351
PENNSYLVANIA		(215) 923-5141
RHODE ISLAND		(401) 331-7433
SOUTH CAROLINA		(803) 268-1722
TENNESSEE		(615) 256-3441
TEXAS	Austin	(512) 474-5321
	Beaumont	(713) 833-5503
	Dallas	(214) 691-1282
	Denton	(817) 387-2914
VIRGINIA		(703) 951-2516
WISCONSIN	Madison	(608) 255-5868
	Milwaukee	(414) 352-4050

PLANNED PARENTHOOD AFFILIATES

PP of Twin Valley Center
4361 Railroad Avenue, Suite G
Pleasanton, Calif. 94566
(415) 462-1950

PP Assn. of Sacramento
Midtown Building, Suite 100
1507 21st Street
Sacramento, Calif. 95814
(916) 446-5034

PP Assn. of San Diego County
1172 Morena Boulevard
San Diego, Calif. 92110
(714) 233-7638

PP of San Francisco
2340 Clay Street, 7th Fl.
San Francisco, Calif. 94115
(415) 567-0870

PP Assn. of Santa Clara County
28 North 16th Street
San Jose, Calif. 95112
(408) 294-2442 or 292-6584

PP Assn. of San Mateo County
373 South Claremont Street
San Mateo, Calif. 94401
(415) 344-6864 or 348-2424

PP Assn. of Marin County
710 C Street, Suite 9
San Rafael, Calif. 94901
(415) 454-0471

PP of Santa Barbara County, Inc.
322 Palm Avenue
Santa Barbara, Calif. 93101
(805) 963-4417

PP of Santa Cruz County
P.O. Box 1196
Santa Cruz, Calif. 95060
(408) 426-5550

PP of Santa Maria
900 West Foster Road
c/o Santa Maria Public Health
Santa Maria, Calif. 93454
(805) 963-4417

PP of San Joaquin County
116 West Willow
Stockton, Calif. 95202
(209) 464-5809

PP of Contra Costa County, Inc.
1291 Oakland Boulevard
Walnut Creek, Calif. 94596
(415) 935-3010

Yolo County Health & Family
   Planning Assn., Inc.
327 College Street, Suite 102
Woodland, Calif. 95695
(916) 666-0707

COLORADO

PP of Boulder
3450 Broadway
Boulder, Colo. 80302
(303) 444-3250

PP of Colorado Springs
722½ South Wahsatch
Colorado Springs, Colo. 80903
(303) 634-3771

Rocky Mountain PP, Inc.
2030 East 20th Avenue
Denver, Colo. 80205
(303) 388-4215

PP of Greeley
155 17th Avenue
Greeley, Colo. 80631
(303) 353-0540

PP of Pueblo
151 Central Main
Pueblo, Colo. 81002
(303) 545-0246

CONNECTICUT

Bridgeport PP
1067 Park Avenue
Bridgeport, Conn. 06604
(203) 366-0664

Danbury PP
240 Main Street
Danbury, Conn. 06810
(203) 743-2446

Hartford PP
293 Farmington Avenue
Hartford, Conn. 06105
(203) 522-6201

Meriden/Wallingford PP
525 Preston Street
Meriden, Conn. 06450
(203) 634-1180

Middlesex PP
60 Crescent Street
Middletown, Conn. 06457
(203) 347-5255

New Britain PP
P.O. Box 292
New Britain, Conn. 06050
(203) 225-9811

PP League of Connecticut, Inc.
406 Orange Street
New Haven, Conn. 06511
(203) 865-6986

Southeastern Chapter, PP
325 Washington Street
Norwich, Conn. 06310
(203) 887-8962

Southern Fairfield PP
259 Main Street
Stamford, Conn. 06901
(203) 327-2722

Northwestern Chapter, PP
189 Litchfield Street
Torrington, Conn. 06790
(203) 489-5500

Waterbury PP
59 Cooke Street
Waterbury, Conn. 06702
(203) 757-1955

Northeastern Chapter, PP
132 Valley Street
Willimantic, Conn. 06226
(203) 432-1500

DELAWARE

Delaware League for PP, Inc.
825 Washington Street
Wilmington, Del. 19801
(302) 655-7293 or 655-8852

DISTRICT OF COLUMBIA

PP of Metropolitan Washington, D.C.
1109 M Street, N.W.
Washington, D.C. 20005
(202) DU 7-8787

FLORIDA

PP of Northeast Florida, Inc.
Universal Marion Building, Suite 1010
21 West Church Street
Jacksonville, Fla. 32202
(904) 354-7796

PP of Central Florida
106 West Central Boulevard
Orlando, Fla. 32801
(305) 843-3434

PP of Southwest Florida
Sarasota Memorial Hospital
P.O. Box 2532
1224 South Tamiami Trail
Sarasota, Fla. 33578
(813) 959-2439

PP—Palm Beach Area
601 Hibiscus Street
West Palm Beach, Fla. 33401
(305) 655-7984

GEORGIA

PP Assn. of the Atlanta Area
118 Marietta Street, N.W.
Atlanta, Ga. 30303
(404) 688-9302

PP of East Central Georgia, Inc.
P.O. Box 3293, Hill Station
Augusta, Ga. 30904
(404) 736-1161

PP Assn. of Chatham County
605 Whittaker Street
Savannah, Ga. 31401
(912) 236-1581

HAWAII

Hawaii PP, Inc.
200 North Vineyard Boulevard
Suite 501
Honolulu, Hawaii 96817
(808) 537-5557

PP of Kauai
2786 Wehe Road
Lihue, Kauai, Hawaii 96766
(808) 537-5557

PP of Maui
2133 Main Street, Room 204
Wailuku, Maui, Hawaii 96793
(808) 537-5557

IDAHO

PP Assn. of Idaho, Inc.
P.O. Box 264
Boise, Idaho 83702
(208) 345-0760

ILLINOIS

PP of McLean County
309 West Market
Bloomington, Ill. 61701
(309) 829-3028

PP Assn. of Champaign County
505 South 5th Street
Champaign, Ill. 61820
(217) 352-7961 or 359-8022

PP Assn.—Chicago Area
185 North Wabash Avenue
Chicago, Ill. 60601
(312) 726-5134

PP of Decatur, Inc.
919 North Water Street
Decatur, Ill. 62526
(217) 429-9211

PP Assn. of the Peoria Area
509 West High Street
Peoria, Ill. 61601
(309) 673-6911

PP of the Springfield Area
801 East Carpenter
Springfield, Ill. 62702
(217) 523-8430

INDIANA

PP Assn. of Monroe County
406 South College Avenue
Bloomington, Ind. 47401
(812) 336-0219

PP of Evansville, Inc.
1610 South Weinback
Evansville, Ind. 47714
(812) 423-6277

PP of Northwest Indiana, Inc.
740 Washington Street
Gary, Ind. 46402
(219) 883-0411

PP Assn. of Indianapolis, Inc.
615 North Alabama Street
Indianapolis, Ind. 46204
(317) 634-8019

PP Assn. of Tippecanoe County
P.O. Box 1114
Lafayette, Ind. 47902
(317) 743-9418

PP of Delaware County
261 Johnston Building
Muncie, Ind. 47305
(317) 282-8011

PP of North Central Indiana
201 South Chapin
South Bend, Ind. 46625
(219) 289-8461

PP of Vigo County
1024 South 6th Street
Terre Haute, Ind. 47807
(812) 232-2683

IOWA

PP of Des Moines County
522 North 3rd Street
Burlington, Iowa 52601
(319) 752-4561

PP of Iowa
851 19th Street
Des Moines, Iowa 50613
(515) 282-2101

PP of Southeast Iowa
927 Exchange Street
Keokuk, Iowa 52632
(319) 524-2759

PP of Henry County
Human Services,
Mental Health Institute
Mt. Pleasant, Iowa 56241
(319) 385-4310

PP Committee of Sioux City
2825 Douglas Street
Sioux City, Iowa 51101
(712) 258-4019

PP of Washington County
309 West 2nd Street
Washington, Iowa 52601
(319) 653-3525

PP of Northeast Iowa
604 Mulberry
Waterloo, Iowa 50703
(319) 235-6243

KANSAS

PP of South Central Kansas
1365 North Custer
Wichita, Kans. 67203
(316) 942-1539

KENTUCKY

Mountain Maternal Health
    League, Inc.
211 Municipal Building
Berea, Ky. 40403
(606) 986-4677

PP of Lexington
331 West 2nd Street
Lexington, Ky. 40507
(606) 255-4913

PP Center, Inc.
843-845 Barret Avenue
Louisville, Ky. 40204
(502) 584-2471

MARYLAND

PP Assn. of Maryland, Inc.
517 North Charles Street
Baltimore, Md. 21201
(301) PL 2-0131

PP of Prince George's County
5101 Pierce Avenue, No. 2
College Park, Md. 20704
(301) 345-5252/3

PP of Montgomery County
11141 Georgia Avenue, Room 420
Wheaton, Md. 20902
(301) 933-2300

MASSACHUSETTS

PP League of Massachusetts
93 Union Street
Newton Centre, Mass. 02159
(617) 332-8750

MICHIGAN

Northern Michigan PP
P.O. Box 624
Alpena, Mich. 49707
(616) 347-4511

Washtenaw County League for PP
313 North 1st Street
Ann Arbor, Mich. 48103
(313) 663-3306

PP Assn. of Southwestern Michigan
997 Agard Street
Benton Harbor, Mich. 49022
(616) 926-6159 or 925-1306

Mecosta County Family Planning
Route #1, Box 261
Big Rapids, Mich. 49307
(616) 345-1197

PP League, Inc.
Professional Plaza Concourse
  Building
3750 Woodward Avenue
Detroit, Mich. 48201
(313) 832-7200

Flint Community PP Assn.
311·East Court Street
Flint, Mich. 48503
(313) 238-3631

PP of Ottawa County
414 Washington Street
Grand Haven, Mich. 49417
(616) 842-8490

PP Assn. of Kent County, Inc.
425 Cherry, S.E.
Grand Rapids, Mich. 49502
(616) 459-3101

PP Assn. of Kalamazoo County
612 Douglas Avenue
Kalamazoo, Mich. 49007
(616) 349-8631

PP League of Monroe County, Inc.
1 East Front Street
Monroe, Mich. 48161
(313) 242-7154

Muskegon Area PP Assn., Inc.
1095 3rd Street
Muskegon, Mich. 49440
(616) 722-2928

Northern Michigan PP Assn., Inc.
603 East Lake Street
Petoskey, Mich. 49770
(616) 347-4511

Traverse City Area PP
717 South Union
Traverse City, Mich. 49684
(616) 946-6910

MINNESOTA

PP Clinic of St. Louis County
504 East 2nd Street
Duluth, Minn. 55585
(612) 722-0833

PP of Mankato
215 North Front Street
Mankato, Minn. 56001
(507) 345-3631

PP of Metropolitan Minneapolis
223 Walker Building
803 Hennepin Avenue
Minneapolis, Minn. 55403
(612) 336-8931

PP of Minnesota, SE Region
116½ South Broadway
Rochester, Minn. 55901
(507) 288-5186

PP of Minnesota, Inc.
Midway Shopping Center
1562 University Avenue
St. Paul, Minn. 55104
(612) 646-9603

PP of St. Paul Metropolitan Area
408 Hamm Building
408 St. Peter Street
St. Paul, Minn. 55102
(612) 224-1361

MISSOURI

PP of Central Missouri
800 North Providence Road, Suite 5
Columbia, Mo. 65201
(314) 443-7255

PP Assn. of Western Missouri/
Kansas
4950 Cherry Street
Kansas City, Mo. 64110
(816) 931-4121

PP of Northeast Missouri
113 East Washington
Kirksville, Mo. 63501
(816) 655-5672

PP of the Central Ozarks
P.O. Box 359
Rolla, Mo. 65401
(314) 364-1509

PP Assn. of St. Louis
4947 Delmar Boulevard
St. Louis, Mo. 63108
(314) 361-6360

PP of Southwest Missouri
430 South Street, Suite 503
Springfield, Mo. 65802
(417) 869-6471

PP of Warrensburg
Route #5, Box #4
Warrensburg, Mo. 64093
(816) 931-4121

MONTANA

PP of Billings
2718 Montana Avenue
Billings, Mont. 59101
(406) 252-2131

NEBRASKA

PP Committee of Nebraska
4155 Dewey Avenue
Omaha, Neb. 68105
(402) 342-2844 or 342-2400

NEVADA

PP of Southern Nevada, Inc.
1380 East Sahara Avenue
Las Vegas, Nev. 89105
(702) 732-9729

PP of Washoe County
505 North Arlington
Reno, Nev. 89503
(702) 322-7372

NEW HAMPSHIRE

PP Assn. of the Upper Valley
14 Parkhurst Street
Lebanon, N.H. 03766
(603) 448-1214

NEW JERSEY

PP of the Greater Camden Area
590 Benson Street
Camden, N.J. 08103
(609) 365-3519

PP of Middlesex County
174 Brower Avenue
Edison, N.J. 08817
(201) 225-2777

PP Center of Bergen County
59 Essex Street
Hackensack, N.J. 07601
(201) 489-1155

PP Assn. of Hudson County
777 Bergen Avenue, Room 218
Jersey City, N.J. 07303
(201) 332-2565

PP Center-Morris Area, Inc.
197 Speedwell
Morristown, N.J. 08960
(201) 539-1364

PP—Essex County
15 William Street
Newark, N.J. 07102
(201) 642-0606

Passaic County PP Center
105 Presidential Boulevard
Riverview Towers, Building #2
Paterson, N.J. 07522
(201) 274-4925

PP of Union County Area, Inc.
234 Park Avenue
Plainfield, N.J. 07060
(201) 756-3736

PP of Monmouth County
141 Bodman Place
Red Bank, N.J. 07701
(201) 842-9300

PP Assn. of the Mercer Area
211 Academy Street
Trenton, N.J. 08618
(609) 599-4881

NEW MEXICO

Bernalillo County PP Assn., Inc.
113 Montclaire, S.E.
Albuquerque, N.M. 87108
(505) 265-3722, Ext. 21

PP of Grant County
Box 214
Fort Bayard, N.M. 88036
(505) 537-3093

Dona Ana County PP Assn.
221 West Griggs Avenue
Las Cruces, N.M. 88001
(505) 524-8516

NEW YORK

PP of Albany
225 Lark Street
Albany, N.Y. 12210
(518) 463-5432

PP of Broome County, Inc.
710 O'Neill Building
Binghamton, N.Y. 13901
(607) 723-8306

PP Center of Buffalo
210 Franklin Street
Buffalo, N.Y. 14202
(716) 853-1771

PP of Ontario County, Inc.
9 North Street
Canandaigua, N.Y. 14424
(315) 394-0310

St. Lawrence County PP Center
95 Main Street
Canton, N.Y. 13617
(315) 386-2441

PP of Nassau County
East Meadow Medical Center
1940 Hempstead Turnpike
East Meadow, N.Y. 11554
(516) 292-8380

PP of the Southern Tier
200 East Market Street
Elmira, N.Y. 14901
(607) 734-3313

Southern Adirondack PP Assn.
11 Little Street
Glens Falls, N.Y. 12801
(518) 792-5148

PP Center of North Suffolk
17 East Carver Street
Huntington, N.Y. 11743
(516) 427-7154

PP of Tompkins County
512 East State Street
Ithaca, N.Y. 14850
(607) 273-1513

Lewis County PP
7552 State Street
Lowville, N.Y. 13367
(315) 376-2741

Franklin County PP
109 East Main Street
Malone, N.Y. 12953
(518) 483-7150

Northern Westchester PP Center
239 Lexington Avenue
Mt. Kisco, N.Y. 10649
(914) 666-6026

Southern Westchester PP Center
16 South 2nd Avenue
Mt. Vernon, N.Y. 10554
(914) 668-7927

PP Center of Orange and
    Sullivan Counties
91 DuBois Street
Newburgh, N.Y. 12550
(914) 562-5748

Margaret Sanger Research Bureau
17 West 16th Street
New York, N.Y. 10010
(212) WA 9-6200

Family Planning Information Service
300 Park Avenue South
New York, N.Y. 10010
(212) 677-3040

PP of New York City, Inc.
300 Park Avenue South
New York, N.Y. 10010
(212) 777-2002

Niagara Assn. for Family
    Planning, Inc.
906 Michigan Avenue
Niagara Falls, N.Y. 14305
(716) 282-1223/4

PP Assn. of Delaware and
    Otsego Counties, Inc.
A.O. Fox Memorial Hospital
1 Norton Avenue
Oneonta, N.Y. 13820

PP of East Suffolk, Inc.
119 North Ocean Avenue
Patchogue, N.Y. 11772
(516) 475-5705

PP of Clinton County
P.O. Box 885
Plattsburgh, N.Y. 12901
(518) 561-4430

Eastern Westchester PP Center
225 Westchester Avenue
Port Chester, N.Y. 10573
(914) 939-1020 or 939-1028

PP League of Dutchess County
85 Market Street
Poughkeepsie, N.Y. 12601
(914) 471-1540

PP League of Rochester and
    Monroe Counties
38 Windsor Street
Rochester, N.Y. 14605
(716) 546-2595

PP League of Schenectady County,
    Inc.
414 Union Street
Schenectady, N.Y. 12305
(518) 374-5353

PP Center of Syracuse, Inc.
1120 East Genessee Street
Syracuse, N.Y. 13210
(315) 475-3193

PP Assn. of the Mohawk Valley, Inc.
11 Devereaux Street
Utica, N.Y. 13501
(315) 724-6146

PP of Northern New York
161 Stone Street
Watertown, N.Y. 13601
(315) 788-8065

PP of Rockland County
37 Village Square
West Nyack, N.Y. 10994
(914) 358-1145

PP of Westchester, Inc.
149 Grand Street
White Plains, N.Y. 10601
(914) 428-7876

Hudson River PP Center
45 Warburton Avenue
Yonkers, N.Y. 10701
(914) 965-1912

NORTH CAROLINA

PP of Western North Carolina
P.O. Box 5641
Asheville, N.C. 28803
(704) 252-1550

PP of Greater Charlotte
1416 East Morehead Street
Charlotte, N.C. 28207
(704) 334-9563

OHIO

PP Assn. of Summit County, Inc.
137 South Main Street, Room 218
Akron, Ohio 44308
(216) 535-2671

PP of Southeast Ohio
8 North Court Street
Security Building, Room 306
Athens, Ohio 45601
(604) 593-3375

PP of Stark County
425 2nd Street, N.W.
Canton, Ohio 44702
(216) 456-7191

PP Assn. of Cincinnati
2406 Auburn Avenue
Cincinnati, Ohio 45219
(513) 721-7635

PP of Cleveland, Inc.
2027 Cornell Road
Cleveland, Ohio 44106
(216) 721-4700

PP Assn. of Columbus
206 East State Street
Columbus, Ohio 43215
(614) 224-8423

PP Assn. of the Miami Valley, Inc.
124 East 3rd Street
Dayton, Ohio
(513) 224-1663

PP Assn. of Crawford County
112 South Market Street
Galion, Ohio 44883
(419) 468-9926

PP Assn. of Butler County
305 South Front Street
Hamilton, Ohio 45011
(513) 893-0451

Maternal Health Assn. of
  Lorain County
1948 Broadway
Lorain, Ohio 44052
(216) 245-4712

PP Assn. of the Mansfield Area
35 North Park Street
Mansfield, Ohio 44902
(419) 525-3075

PP Assn. of East Central Ohio
7 North 1st Street
Newark, Ohio 43055
(614) 345-7445

Family Planning Assn. of Lake and
  Geauga Counties
1499 Mentor Avenue
Painesville Shopping Center,
  The Arcade
Painesville, Ohio 44077

PP of West Central Ohio
401 North Plum Street
Springfield, Ohio 45504
(513) 325-7349

PP League of Toledo
217 15th Street
Toledo, Ohio 43624
(419) 246-3651

PP of Ashland-Wayne Counties
353 Pine Street
Wooster, Ohio 44691
(419) 262-4866

PP of Mahoning Valley
502 Executive Building
125 West Commerce Street
Youngstown, Ohio 44503
(216) 746-5641

OKLAHOMA

PP Assn. of Oklahoma City
740 Culbertson Drive
Oklahoma City, Okla. 73105
(405) 528-2157

PP Assn. of Tulsa
1615 East 12th Street
Tulsa, Okla. 74120
(918) 587-1101

OREGON

PP of Benton County, Inc.
Family Planning Clinic
610 Van Buren
Corvallis, Ore. 97330
(503) 753-3348

PP Assn. of Lane County
142 East 14th Street
Eugene, Ore. 97401
(503) 344-9411 or 344-1611

PP of Jackson County
Professional Plaza, Suite 11
650 Royal Avenue
Medford, Ore. 97501
(503) 773-8285

PP Assn., Inc.
1200 Southeast Morrison
Portland, Ore. 97214
(503) 287-1189

PENNSYLVANIA

PP Assn. of Lehigh County
33 North 5th Street
Allentown, Pa. 18101
(215) 439-1033

PP Assn. of Bucks County
Professional Center
Bath Road and Route 13
Bristol, Pa. 19007
(215) 788-4121

PP of Easton
415 Valley Street
Easton, Pa. 18042
(215) 252-3844

Monroe County PP Assn.
P.O. Box 76
East Stroudsburg, Pa. 18301
(717) 421-4000

PP Assn. of Erie County
G. Daniel Baldwin Building,
  Suites 818-820
1005 State Street
Erie, Pa. 16507
(814) 453-6473

PP of Lancaster
37 South Lime Street
Lancaster, Pa. 17601
(717) 394-3575

PP Assn. of Southeastern
Pennsylvania
1402 Spruce Street
Philadelphia, Pa. 19102
(215) 732-5880

PP Center of Pittsburgh, Inc.
526 Penn Avenue
Pittsburgh, Pa. 15222
(412) 281-9502

PP Center of Berks County
48 South 4th Street
Reading, Pa. 19602
(215) 376-8061

PP Organization of
Lackawanna County
316 North Washington Avenue
Scranton, Pa. 18503
(717) 344-2626

PP of Mercer County
Boyle Building
149 East State Street
Sharon, Pa. 16146
(412) 347-1402

PP of Chester County
134 North Church Street
West Chester, Pa. 19380
(215) 692-8080

PP Assn. of Luzerne County
Kirby Health Center Annex
63 North Franklin Street
Wilkes-Barre, Pa. 18701
(717) 824-8921

PP Committee of York County
Visiting Nurses Assn. Building
218 East Market Street
York, Pa. 17403
(717) 843-7151

RHODE ISLAND

PP of Rhode Island
46 Aborn Street
Providence, R.I. 02903
(401) 421-9620

SOUTH CAROLINA

PP of Aiken County
P.O. Box 277
Clearwater, S.C. 29822
(803) 593-9283

PP of Central South Carolina, Inc.
2014 Washington Street
Columbia, S.C. 29201
(803) 256-4908

TENNESSEE

PP Assn. of Knox County
114 Dameron Avenue, N.W.
Knoxville, Tenn. 37917
(615) 524-7487

Memphis PP Assn., Inc.
Exchange Building, Suite 1700
9 North 2nd Street
Memphis, Tenn. 38105

PP Assn. of Nashville
814 Church Street
Nashville, Tenn. 37203
(615) 255-1149

PP Assn. of the Southern Mountains
P.O. Box 88
Oak Ridge, Tenn. 37830
(615) 483-0283

TEXAS

Panhandle PP Assn.
604 West 8th Street
Amarillo, Tex. 79101
(806) 372-8731 or 372-8732

PP Center of Austin
1300 Sabine Street
Austin, Tex. 78701
(512) 472-7311

PP of Cameron County
Security Building, Room 307
Brownsville, Tex. 78520
(512) 546-9445

South Texas PP Center
2206 Crews
Corpus Christi, Tex. 78405
(512) 884-4352

PP of Northeast Texas
2727 Oak Lawn, Suite 228
Dallas, Tex. 75219
(214) 522-0290

PP of Val Verde County
200 Bridge Street
Del Rio, Tex. 78840
(512) 775-4311

PP Center of El Paso
214 West Franklin Street
El Paso, Tex. 79901
(915) 542-1919

PP Center of Fort Worth
614 West 1st Street
Fort Worth, Tex. 76102
(817) 332-9101

PP of Houston
3601 Fannin
Houston, Tex. 77004
(713) 522-3976

PP Assn. of Chaparral County
117 South 5th Street
Kingsville, Tex. 78363
(512) 592-1831

PP of Webb County, Inc.
2000 San Jorge
Laredo, Tex. 78040
(512) 723-5519

PP of Caldwell County
201 West Market Street
Lockhart, Tex. 78644
(512) 398-5412

PP Center of Lubbock
P.O. Box 6193
Lubbock, Tex. 79413
(806) 795-7123

PP Assn. of Hidalgo County
P.O. Box 244
1201 Conway Avenue
Mission, Tex. 78572
(512) JU 5-4575

Permian Basin PP, Inc.
American Bank of Commerce
    Building, Suite 401
Odessa, Tex. 79760
(915) 563-2530

PP Center of San Angelo
122 West 2nd Street
San Angelo, Tex. 76901
(915) 655-3748

PP Center of San Antonio
106 Warren Street
San Antonio, Tex. 78212
(512) 227-2227

PP of Central Texas
1121 Ross Street
Waco, Tex. 76706
(817) 754-2307

UTAH

PP of Utah
1212 South State Street
Salt Lake City, Utah 84116
(801) 363-4471

VERMONT

Barre Family Planning Center
24 Spaulding Street
Barre, Vt. 05641
(802) 476-6696

Brattleboro Family Planning Center
21 Elliott Street
Brattleboro, Vt. 05301
(802) 257-0153

PPA of Vermont
19 Church Street
Burlington, Vt. 05401
(802) 862-9637

Morrisville Birth Planning Clinic
Box 35
Johnson, Vt. 05656
(802) 888-3162

Addison County Birth
   Planning Clinic
26 Main Street
Middlebury, Vt. 05753
(802) 388-2027

Rutland Birth Planning Center
46½ Center Street
Rutland, Vt. 05701
(802) 775-1001

Franklin County Birth
   Planning Center
48 North Main Street
St. Albans, Vt. 05478
(802) 527-7392

St. Johnsbury Family
   Planning Center
79 Railroad Street
St. Johnsbury, Vt. 05819
(802) 748-8194

Family Planning Center
2 Summer Street
Springfield, Vt. 05156
(802) 885-4701

VIRGINIA

PP of Northern Virginia
5827 Columbia Pike
Falls Church, Va. 22041
(703) 820-3335

PP of Norfolk, Inc.
Norfolk Public Health Center
401 Colley Avenue, Room 113
Norfolk, Va. 23507
(703) 625-5591

Virginia League for PP
2009 Monument Avenue
Richmond, Va. 23220
(702) 358-4919

WASHINGTON

PP of Whatcom County
P.O. Box 4
Bellingham, Wash. 98225
(206) 734-9095

PP of Snohomish County
1508 Hewitt Street
Everett, Wash. 98201
(206) 259-0096

PP Center of Seattle
202 16th Avenue, South
Seattle, Wash. 98144
(206) 329-3625 or 329-2450

PP of Spokane
412 Hutton Building
South 9 Washington
Spokane, Wash. 99204
(509) 747-5108

PP of Pierce County
4002 South M Street
Tacoma, Wash. 98408
(206) GR 5-5123

Center for Family Planning
329 South 2nd Street
Walla Walla, Wash. 99362
(509) 529-3570

PP Assn. of Yakima County
208 North 3rd Avenue
Yakima, Wash. 98901
(509) 248-3625

WEST VIRGINIA

PP Assn. of Parkersburg
P.O. Box 5222
Vienna, West Va. 26101
(304) 295-5841

WISCONSIN

PP of Green Bay
Bellin Building, Room 206
130 East Walnut Street
Green Bay, Wisc. 54301
(414) 432-0031

PP of Kenosha
5204 70th Street
Kenosha, Wisc. 53140
(414) 657-6211

PP of Wisconsin
1135 West State Street
Milwaukee, Wisc. 53202
(412) 271-8181

Index

145